LAW AND ETHICS

for Pharmacy Technicians

LAW AND ETHICS

for Pharmacy Technicians

Jahangir Moini, MD, MPH, CPhT
Professor and Former Director
Allied Health Sciences

Pharmacy Technician Program
Everest University
Melbourne, Florida

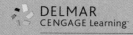

DELMAR
CENGAGE Learning

Australia • Brazil • Japan • Korea • Mexico • Singapore • Spain • United Kingdom • United States

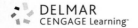

Law and Ethics for Pharmacy Technicians
Jahangir Moini, MD, MPH, CPhT

Vice President, Career and Professional
Editorial: David Garza

Director of Learning Solutions:
Matthew Kane

Acquisitions Editor: Tari Broderick

Managing Editor: Marah Bellegarde

Senior Product Manager: Darcy M. Scelsi

Editorial Assistant: Anthony Souza

Vice President, Career and Professional
Marketing: Jennifer McAvey

Marketing Manager: Kristin McNary

Marketing Coordinator: Erica Ropitzky

Production Director: Carolyn Miller

Content Project Management:
Pre-Press PMG

Senior Art Director: Jack Pendleton

For product information and technology assistance, contact us at
Cengage Learning Customer & Sales Support, 1-800-354-9706
For permission to use material from this text or product,
submit all requests online at **www.cengage.com/permissions**
Further permissions questions can be e-mailed to
permissionrequest@cengage.com

Library of Congress Control Number: 2009925008

ISBN-13: 978-1-4283-1102-2

ISBN-10: 1-4283-1102-5

Delmar Cengage Learning
5 Maxwell Drive
Clifton Park, NY 12065-2919
USA

Cengage Learning is a leading provider of customized learning solutions with office locations around the globe, including Singapore, the United Kingdom, Australia, Mexico, Brazil, and Japan. Locate your local office at: **international.cengage.com/region**

Cengage Learning products are represented in Canada by Nelson Education, Ltd.

To learn more about Delmar, visit **www.cengage.com/delmar**

Purchase any of our products at your local college store or at our preferred online store www.ichapters.com

Printed in the United States of America
3 4 5 6 7 13 12 11 10 09

Dedication

This book is dedicated to

My wife Hengameh, and daughters

Mahkameh and Morvarid.

Contents

Acknowledgements

The author would like to acknowledge the following individuals for their time and efforts in aiding him with their contributions to this book.

Michael Edwards, PharmD
Corporate Director of Pharmacy
Health First
Melbourne, Florida

Norman Tomaka, CRPh, LHCRM
President and Chairman of the Executive Board
Florida Pharmacy Association and Pharmacist Consultant
Melbourne, Florida

Greg Vadimsky, Pharmacy Technician
Melbourne, Florida

REVIEWERS

The author also would like to thank the following reviewers.

Helen A. Batchelder, CPhT
Rassmusen
Minneapolis, Minnesota

Donald Becker, PhD
San Jacinto College
Houston, Texas

Jodie Corwin, CPhT
Tri-State Business Institute
Erie, Pennsylvania

Michael Ellis, CPhT
Trinity College
Vallejo, California

Marcy May, MAEd, CPhT, PhTR
Virginia College
Austin, Texas

Michelle McCranie, CPhT, AAS
Ogeechee Technical College
Statesboro, Georgia

Michelle Miller, PharmD, R.Ph
Kirkwood Community College
Ely, Iowa

James J. Mizner, Jr., RPh, MBA
ACT College
Arlington, Virginia

Philip D. Penrod, Jr., BS, AA.AA, CPhT
Everest University
Tampa, Florida

Preface

INTRODUCTION

This book is designed as a thorough overview of law and ethics in the pharmacy. It reviews federal and state laws and regulations that affect pharmacy technicians, pharmacists, and other pharmacy employees. Special attention is paid to the Controlled Substances Act and the resultant activities of the Food and Drug Administration (FDA) and the Drug Enforcement Agency (DEA). The text emphasizes the importance of ensuring that each patient receives the highest quality care possible. It is the responsibility of the pharmacy technician to assist the pharmacist in respecting the rights of every patient and in providing services that strictly adhere to federal and state laws, as well as the ethical standards of the industry.

ORGANIZATION OF CONTENT

This book focuses on the foundation of law and ethics, federal laws, and state laws affecting pharmacy practice. The Appendices cover diverse topics, including medication errors, pharmacy technician duties and tasks, state boards of pharmacy and requirements, professional organizations, and the United States Pharmacopoeia / National Formulary.

FEATURES

Each chapter contains an outline of the key topics, a list of key terms (which are **bolded** in the chapter text), and objectives that the student must be able to meet upon completion of the reading. Following this is a scenario relevant to each chapter, entitled "Setting the Scene," which includes critical thinking questions to encourage deeper understanding of real-life situations. The answers to these questions are provided near the end of each chapter.

Overviews serve to introduce the student to the key concepts of each chapter. "Focus On" features highlight interesting key points of knowledge. "What Would You Do?" and "You Be the Judge" scenarios offer further realism to the text by providing actual case study-type situations to consider. Accurate tables focus on legal and ethical information that must be fully understood in order to master each chapter's content. Certain chapters contain figures that show legal forms and other paperwork. Chapter summaries serve to reinforce the chapter content and focus on key ideas from the text.

At the end of each chapter, review questions are given which help the student to test the knowledge they have gained from their reading. The questions are given in a variety of formats to encourage more complete comprehension and include case studies. Internet sites are listed to provide avenues for further reference and learning beyond the text. Book references for sources used in each chapter follow. The answer key to each chapter's review questions can be found near the end of the book.

INSTRUCTOR SUPPLEMENT

The Instructor Resource to Accompany Law and Ethics for Pharmacy Technicians is a CD-ROM containing the following:

- A Testbank in Examview containing 600 multiple-choice questions with rationales that explain the correct answers in detail. These questions are designed to be similar to those found on the PTCB exam.
- PowerPoint presentations for each chapter.
- An Instructor Manual that features lecture outlines, teaching strategies, lists of legal cases, and sources for these cases.
- Additional Case Studies to be used in class or to assign as homework

About the Author

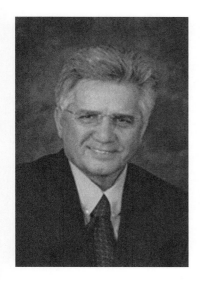

Dr. Moini was assistant professor at Tehran University School of Medicine for 9 years teaching medical and allied health students. The author is a professor and former director (for 15 years) of allied health programs at Everest University. Dr. Moini established, for the first time, the associate degree program for pharmacy technicians in 2000 at EU's Melbourne campus. For 5 years, he was the director of the pharmacy technician program. He also established several other new allied health programs for EU. As a physician and instructor for the past 35 years, he believes that pharmacy technicians should be skillful with various types of compounding, and have confidence in their duties and responsibilities in order to prevent medication errors.

Dr. Moini is actively involved in teaching and helping students to prepare for service in various health professions, including the roles of pharmacy technicians, medical assistants, and nurses. He worked with the Brevard County Health Department as an epidemiologist and health educator consultant for 18 years, offering continuing education courses and keeping nurses up-to-date on the latest developments related to pharmacology, medications errors, immunizations, and other important topics. He has been an internationally published author of various allied health books since 1999.

SECTION I

THE FOUNDATION OF LAW AND ETHICS

Introduction to Law

OUTLINE

OBJECTIVES

Upon completion of this chapter, the reader should be able to:

1. Explain why knowledge of the law is important to pharmacy technicians.
2. Identify the sources of law.
3. Define statutory law.
4. Differentiate between criminal law and civil law.
5. Explain tort law.
6. Describe the U.S. court system.
7. Explain the statute of limitations.
8. List the four elements necessary to prove negligence and explain them.
9. Explain unintentional negligence.
10. Define malpractice as it relates to pharmacy technicians.

KEY TERMS

Administrative law – The body of law governing the administrative agencies (e.g., Occupational Safety and Health Administration or the Department of Public Health) that have been created by Congress or by state legislatures.

Appeal – A legal process in which a case is brought to a higher court to review the decision of a lower court.

Case law – A system of law based on judges' decisions and legal precedents rather than on statutes; in this system, judges can interpret statutory law or apply common law.

Common law – A system of law derived from the decisions of judges rather than from constitutions or statutes.

Contract law – A system of law that pertains to agreements between two or more parties.

Criminal law – The body of law that defines criminal offenses against the public.

Felony – An offense punishable by imprisonment or death in a state or federal prison for more than one year.

Jurisdiction – The power and authority given to a court to hear a case and to make a judgment.

Law – A rule of conduct or procedure established by custom, agreement, or authority.

Legal precedent – A legal principle created by a court decision that provides an example for judges deciding similar issues later.

Legislative law – A law that is prescribed by legislative enactments; also known as statutory law.

Malfeasance – The execution of an unlawful or improper act.

Malpractice – Professional misconduct or demonstration of an unreasonable lack of skill with the result of injury, loss, or damage to the patient.

Misdemeanor – Crimes punishable by fine or by imprisonment in a facility other than a prison for less than one year.

Misfeasance – The improper performance of an act.

Negligence – A type of unintentional tort alleged when one may have performed or failed to perform an act that a reasonable person would or would not have done in similar circumstances.

Nonfeasance – The failure to act when there is a duty to act, as a reasonably prudent person would in similar circumstances.

Statute of limitations – That period of time established by state law during which a lawsuit or criminal proceeding may be filed.

Statutory law – A law that is prescribed by legislative enactments; also known as legislative law.

Tort – A private wrong or injury, other than a breach of contract, for which the court will provide a remedy.

SETTING THE SCENE

A patient brought a prescription to a pharmacy for a sulfa drug that was prescribed by her physician. The patient is allergic to sulfa drugs, a fact that was noted in the written medical record located in the physician's office. However, the medical records assistant did not transcribe the allergy note into the computerized patient record. The pharmacy technician dispensed the drug because there was no information about the patient's sulfa drug allergy included in the computerized patient record. The technician did not ask the patient if she had any drug allergies. The pharmacist signed off and approved the dispensing of the drug. After taking one dose of the sulfa drug, the patient had a severe allergic reaction that ultimately led to her death. The patient's family filed a civil suit against both the pharmacist and the physician for negligence.

Critical Thinking

- What should the pharmacy technician have done to best benefit the patient in this situation?

- Was it appropriate for the patient's family to sue the pharmacist?

- If criminal charges were to be filed, what would be the possible outcomes that may affect the pharmacist, the physician, and the pharmacy technician?

OVERVIEW

Every job, profession, and career has a distinct vocabulary and a set of professional standards and regulations. Once familiar with the vocabulary, rules, and regulations, the ideas, concepts, and structure of the job become understandable. The practice of pharmacy is regulated at both the federal and state levels. Pharmacists and pharmacy technicians need to have a clear understanding of the laws and regulations related to their field of practice. If these laws and regulations are not understood and not followed, the consequences to the consumer of pharmaceutical products could be life-threatening.

ROLE OF LAW

Law includes statutes, rules, and regulations that govern people, behaviors, relationships, and interactions with society and with state and federal governments. Law provides order for the resolution of conflicts between individuals, corporations, states, and other entities. The goal of law is to protect the health, safety, and welfare of individual citizens. Law provides guidelines for resolutions of disputes in a fair and safe manner.

Although based on solid and long-held beliefs, customs, and principles, the law is always growing and evolving to meet the changes, challenges, and constantly occurring shifts of society. This can be evidenced by the history of drug laws in the United States. In the 1800s and early 1900s there was no regulation or control over medicinals. Any product or substance could claim health benefits and medicinal effects. As a result, contamination of products occurred that led to injury to the consumer, and products were used that could lead to addiction. In response to these circumstances, laws such as the Pure Food and Drug Act (enacted to ensure accurate labeling and the purity of marketed foods and drugs) were passed. Some of these laws, such as the Food, Drug, and Cosmetic Act of 1938, resulted in the establishment of agencies such as the Food and Drug Administration (FDA), which regulates food and drugs along with the proper labeling of their contents. As time went on, deficiencies in legislation were identified and additional legislation was enacted to continue to improve pharmacological products in the United States. For instance, laws were enacted to make certain substances illegal for public use or to limit their types of usage. Fine tuning of laws continues today as the need arises.

SOURCES OF LAW

Law is developed from a variety of sources. The most important source of law is the United States Constitution. In the United States, law was originally derived from common law as defined by England.

The four sources of law include:

- The Constitution and the Bill of Rights – Constitutional law
- The Legislative Branch of the Government – Statutory or legislative law
- The Executive Branch of the Government – Administrative law
- The Judicial Branch of the Government – Common or case law

Constitutional Law

The Constitution is the foundation of the law in the United States and grants certain powers to the federal government. The states have the power to regulate health care through the powers of protecting the health, safety, and welfare of each state's citizens. The states regulate nurses, pharmacists, physicians, physical therapists, chiropractors, and other licensed health-care providers through state boards and licensure.

Individuals are guaranteed certain fundamental freedoms by the Constitution and the Bill of Rights. These include the fundamental rights to privacy, freedom of speech, religion, equal protection, and due process. The Health Insurance Portability and Accountability Act (HIPAA) is legislation that protects the consumer's right to privacy. HIPAA will be discussed more thoroughly in Chapter 5.

Focus On...

The Constitution and Bill of Rights

To further explore these important historical documents visit http://www.archives.gov. Search for the Charters of Freedom, the Constitution, or the Bill of Rights. Read and explore these important documents as originally written.

Statutory or Legislative Law

Statutory law, also known as **legislative law**, consists of rules (laws) enacted by federal and state legislative bodies. The judicial branch (or system) interprets statutory law. Earlier decisions are considered precedent and are binding on all lower courts.

Statutes are laws enacted by legislatures. Statutes start as bills (at the federal or state levels) and may become laws or be vetoed by governors or presidents. When they are signed, these laws can be repealed (revoked), revised (modified), amended (changed or improved), or superseded (replaced) by legislatures. The courts can review them for application, constitutionality, interpretation, and other legal questions.

Municipal ordinances are laws passed by city governments as allowed by state statutes. If these ordinances are violated, the offender will be legally opposed by the city that enacted the ordinances.

Administrative Law

The executive branch can introduce laws or veto laws that are proposed by the legislative branch, and also enforce laws and propose and establish agencies. Congress or individual state legislatures may create administrative agencies. These agencies can enact rules and regulations that become **administrative law**. The Occupational Safety and Health Administration (OSHA) is one such agency whose rules apply to most workplaces, including health-care facilities and the pharmacy. Similarly, state Departments of Public Health (DPH) regulate health-care workplaces, including nursing homes, hospitals, and other facilities.

Focus On...

Executive Orders

Executive orders are those that are issued by the President without congressional approval, and have the force of law upon government agencies without actually being laws.

Common or Case Law

Common law, what is now known as **case law**, was developed by judges in Europe over many centuries. Originally coming from England, it was practiced for the first time in America by the Pilgrims and other settlers of this country. Since then, every state's courts have decided various cases that fall under the description of common law. Case law, which began with common law, is law that is set by legal precedent. Common law was derived from laws that were not even written down, and were based on the customs and traditions of the people. Eventually, court decisions were written down and judges often referred to them to help make their own case decisions. These written cases were used as legal precedents. Today, legal precedents are the rule of law, and apply to future cases. Precedents can only be changed by the court that originally decided a case, or by a higher court.

DIVISIONS OF LAW

In the United States, the legal system divides laws into three categories: criminal law, civil law, and administrative law. Criminal laws are enforced by representatives of the state against persons or corporations. In civil law, a plaintiff (injured party) may bring suit against an alleged defendant (wrongdoer). Administrative law focuses on the regulations set forth and enforced by governmental administrative agencies.

Criminal Law

Criminal law is concerned with violations against society based on criminal statutes or codes. State or federal governments may impose monetary fines, imprisonment, or even death in certain circumstances for violations of criminal law. Misdemeanors are lesser crimes usually punishable by fines and/or imprisonment of less than 1 year (for example, traffic violations, thefts under a certain dollar amount, or attempted burglary). Felonies are punishable by much larger fines, and imprisonment for more than 1 year or in some states punishable by death (for example, rape, murder, domestic violence, or child abuse).

Many states hold that certain felony convictions are grounds for revoking licenses to practice in the health-care field. Practice without a license, falsifying information when obtaining a license, failing to provide life support for those who are terminally ill, and patient abuse are all examples of crimes that may result in criminal prosecutions. The state or federal government may pose criminal charges against those who violate written criminal codes or statutes.

Focus On...

Criminal Law

Criminal law involves crimes against the state.

> **What Would You Do?**
>
> *Brian has had three traffic violations in the past three months. He has also been charged with domestic violence against his girlfriend. You are the pharmacist for whom Brian works, and you are aware of some of these events. One day, you hear him harassing another worker until an argument breaks out. Brian becomes very agitated. Knowing his background, what would you do in this situation?*

Civil Law

Civil wrongs are often called torts. A **tort** is an injury to a person – physical or non-physical – by another person. The person causing the injury is legally responsible for his or her actions. The injury may be intentional or unintentional. "Tort" is an Anglo-French word meaning "wrong." Torts may include cases of assault (in general, the threat of violence), battery (contact in a manner that may cause bodily harm), fraud, libel, negligence, slander, theft, trespassing, and even wrongful death. Tort law often results in civil lawsuits.

Most civil law cases against health-care workers are for **malpractice** (professional misconduct or negligence) or **negligence** (failure to exercise reasonable care). Penalties in civil law are almost completely monetary in nature, in an attempt to make the injured or wronged person "whole" again. Individuals or entities may bring civil cases against other individuals or entities for harm involving contracts, labor, privacy, or tort issues.

Intentional torts are those that are committed willfully. The injured party may seek a civil case against the person who committed the tort against them. Intentional torts include assault, battery, false imprisonment, fraud, libel, slander, trespassing, and invasion of privacy. Some intentional torts may also be prosecuted as crimes in additional court cases. Unintentional torts are those that are committed accidentally. For example, when a pharmacy technician fails to verify accurate information, and a patient receives a medication that is less effective than intended, an unintentional tort has occurred. Negligence, malpractice, and product liability are examples of unintentional torts.

Contract Law

Contract law pertains to agreements between two or more parties. In a contract, each of the concerned parties makes agreements to do or not to do certain things. Contracts are legally binding exchanges of promises. The term "contract law" is based on the Latin phrase "*pacta sunt servanda,*" which means, "pacts must be kept."

THE U.S. COURT SYSTEM

There are several levels of courts in each state. Local courts usually deal with civil and criminal cases that do not exceed certain punitive sums that are established by the legislature. The next level is a court with general jurisdiction. This includes any major trial court that has broad powers. Often, cases of negligence, malpractice, elder abuse, and other civil wrongs are tried at this level. Major crimes are also prosecuted in these courts.

A court must have **jurisdiction** over any case that it tries, whether *in personam* (over the person) or *in rem* (over the thing or property). Major trial courts' jurisdiction is based on county lines or similar divisions and the people within those divisions.

When a trial is completed or a case is final in a court of general jurisdiction or one of the specific courts, the case may be appealed to a higher court (usually called an *appeals court*). **Appeals** may only raise issues of law and facts (as found by a jury or a judge in a previous case) for review in consideration for overturning the previous ruling. If decided by an appeals court, the appellate decision is binding on all lower courts in the state if no further appeals are taken.

The top court of a state is usually called its *supreme court*, with the only recourse after that being the *United States Supreme Court*. However, the U.S. Supreme Court chooses to hear only a few cases as determined by vote of at least four justices. The cases chosen are usually the most important and consequential cases that have been petitioned. Once the Supreme Court makes its decision and tries a case, the decision is binding on all state and federal courts.

Focus On...

The Supreme Court

Supreme Court Justices are appointed by the President of the United States and approved by the Senate. An appointment to the Supreme Court is a lifetime appointment.

Some cases may be tried in a federal district court. These courts hear cases that raise issues of federal law, or those involving parties from different states with an amount in controversy that exceeds $75,000.

THE DIFFERENCES BETWEEN FEDERAL LAW AND STATE LAW

Neither federal nor state courts are completely independent of each other. Many federal and state laws interact. Federal courts handle crimes under statutes that have been enacted by Congress. Table 1-1 outlines the types of cases related to pharmacy that are handled in federal and state courts.

Individual states have the authority to enact legislation in any area in which Congress has enacted legislation as long as no conflicts between the two laws are created. If a conflict exists, federal law outweighs state law and must be enforced. A conflict may exist if a state law is less strict then the federal law and following the state law would be in violation of the federal law. If, however, the state law is stricter than the federal law, then no conflict with the federal law exists and the state law would be followed without being in violation of the federal law.

TABLE 1-1 Courts Handling Specific Pharmacy-Related Cases

Federal	State	Both
Interstate and international trade/commerce cases	Cases involving state laws or regulations	Crimes that can be punished under federal or state law
Bankruptcy cases	Most private contract disputes	Class action cases
Disputes between individual states	Most trade or professional regulation cases	Environmental regulation cases
	Most professional malpractice cases	
	Most business law cases	
	Most personal injury cases	
	Most worker-injury cases	

Adapted from www.uscourts.gov/outreach/courtjurisdiction.pdf

Statute of Limitations

The **statute of limitations** is the period of time established by state law during which a lawsuit or criminal proceeding may be filed. Statute of limitations varies by state and by the type of legal claim. Pharmacy technicians must understand the specific laws and statutes of their state. Statutory time limits apply to many legal actions, including collections, wrongful death claims, and medical malpractice. In filing professional negligence suits, the statute of limitations is generally from 1 to 8 years, with 2 years being most common. Therefore, patients cannot file negligence lawsuits against physicians if this designated length of time has expired.

The most common occurrences for marking the beginning of a statutory period are:

- On the day that the negligence was allegedly committed

- When the resulting injury from the alleged negligence was actually discovered, or should have been discovered, by a reasonably alert patient

- The day the patient/physician relationship ended, or the day of last medical treatment in a series

Specific statutory time limits may be found in state codes, online, and in most libraries.

Negligence

Negligence is defined as delivery of care that is below the expected standard. The unintentional tort of negligence is the most common liability in medicine. It usually means any deviation from the accepted medical standard of care that causes patient injury.

All medical professional liability claims are classified as either:

- **Malfeasance** – The performance of a totally wrongful and unlawful act, such as the prescribing of medications by a person who is not licensed to do so

- **Misfeasance** – The performance of a lawful act in an illegal or improper manner, such as not using sterile technique when preparing an IV, and therefore causing a resultant infection

- **Nonfeasance** – The failure to act when one should, such as failing to scan a bar code on a package

There are four elements that must occur to prove a health-care professional guilty of negligence. The "four D's of negligence" include:

- Duty – The health-care professional owed a duty of care to the accuser
- Dereliction – The health-care professional breached the duty of care to the patient
- Direct cause – The breach of care was a direct cause of the patient's injury
- Damages – There is a legally recognizable injury to the patient, with the burden of proof on the plaintiff (the patient's attorney must present evidence of the four D's of negligence)

You Be the Judge

Pamela is a pharmacy technician who recently prepared eyedrops for a patient with glaucoma. The patient used the eyedrops per the enclosed instructions, but experienced no positive effects, and, after 1 week, continued experiencing minor but continuing visual impairment. The patient went back to her physician and complained about the eyedrops she had used. He checked the eyedrops, finding out that they were long past their expiration date. In your judgment, what would the possible consequences be for Pamela since the expiration date had not been checked before the medication was dispensed by the pharmacist? In addition, what would happen to the pharmacist because of this error?

MALPRACTICE

When a patient is treated in a manner that is improper or negligent, the pharmacist or pharmacy technician may be sued for malpractice. Negligent behavior that results in injury, damage, loss, or death is referred to as *malpractice*. It is important to understand that malpractice also governs unethical practices. Malpractice lawsuits have increased dramatically. Malpractice insurance covers a wide variety of health-care practitioners, including doctors, nurses, pharmacists, and even pharmacy technicians.

Professional liability insurance protects against suits being brought against pharmacists or pharmacy technicians for malpractice. Though amounts of coverage vary, plans are available (for example, for pharmacists and technicians) that pay $1 million per claim up to three claims per year. These policies are able to cover property loss or damage, personal injury, death, and even legal costs.

Having adequate schooling, certification, licensure, registration, and insurance coverage, according to the requirements of state law, all help to protect against legal action. Pharmacists and pharmacy technicians may take specific steps that will help to protect against errors and acts that could lead to legal actions being taken against them. These steps are as follows:

- Always communicate effectively, accurately, and correctly – always be straightforward, honest, and descriptive in communications; ask patients to reflect to you their understanding of what you have told them.

- Conversations and documents must be thorough and complete, covering all necessary information that will promote a good patient outcome – every piece of information that affects the patient's health and well-being must be included in communications and patient records.

- Being concise is also important – anything not focused on the patient's health and outcome is not required to be included in conversation or documents; wordiness and restating of information is not necessary; the patient record should not include information unnecessary to patient care.

- Verbal and written communication must remain consistently handled; behaviors and patterns of communication must remain relatively the same for all patients so that the focus on good patient care may be uniform and maintained for all patients.

- All verbal or written wording of information must be cautiously presented, avoiding terms that may be confused or may represent the intentions of the pharmacy staff; suggestions for future patient-care methods may be made, but should not be demands or warnings; considerations that may be required, as well as suggestions regarding care, should be indicated in a positive manner.

SUMMARY

The practice of dispensing drugs is subject to many laws and regulations. Both state and federal laws affect the profession and practice of pharmacy. Pharmacy technicians must be familiar with terminology, concepts, and the structure of their jobs; this includes knowledge of the legal issues surrounding pharmacy. A pharmacy technician should know types and sources of law, the court system, and relevant statutes of limitations. Negligence is the most common liability in medicine that also affects pharmacists and technicians.

Laws that are broken in this profession are punishable by monetary fines and imprisonment.

SETTING THE SCENE

The following discussion and responses relate to the opening "Setting the Scene" scenario:

- The pharmacy technician should have double-checked with the patient to find if she had any allergies to sulfa drugs.

- It was appropriate for the patient's family to sue the pharmacist since he has supreme responsibility for the welfare of every patient to whom he dispenses.

- If the patient's family wins this case, the pharmacist and the physician may be at risk for additional administrative or criminal actions resulting in fines, imprisonment, and the loss of their licenses to practice.

REVIEW QUESTIONS

Multiple Choice

1. Treating a patient in a manner that is improper or negligent is an example of:

   A. misfeasance
   B. misdemeanor
   C. malpractice
   D. remedy

2. Which of the following is a type of punishment for a felony?

   A. imprisonment for more than one year
   B. large fines
   C. death
   D. all of the above

3. Local courts usually deal with which of the following types of cases?

   A. civil law
   B. criminal law
   C. both A and B
   D. none of the above

4. Very few cases are chosen to be heard by which of the following?

    A. local court
    B. state court
    C. court of general jurisdiction
    D. U.S. Supreme Court

5. *Statutory law* refers to laws enacted by:

    A. state legislatures
    B. federal legislatures
    C. both state and federal legislatures
    D. the President

6. The statute of limitations is generally from 1 year to:

    A. 2 years
    B. 4 years
    C. 6 years
    D. 8 years

7. The "four D's of negligence" include each of the following except:

    A. Direct cause
    B. Depth of cause
    C. Derelict
    D. Damages

8. After a trial is completed or a case is final in a court, the case may be:

    A. stopped
    B. waived
    C. appealed
    D. none of the above

9. Which of the following is a crime that may result in criminal prosecution?

    A. practicing without a license
    B. falsifying information when obtaining a license
    C. failure to provide reasonable care
    D. all of the above

10. Cases of negligence, malpractice, and elder abuse are tried at which of the following levels of courts?

    A. appeals court
    B. general jurisdiction court
    C. State Supreme Court
    D. U.S. Supreme Court

11. The failure to act when one should is termed:

    A. nonfeasance
    B. noninvasive
    C. misfeasance
    D. malfeasance

12. Professional liability insurance protects pharmacy technicians against which of the following?

    A. constitutional law
    B. common law
    C. tort law
    D. lawsuits

13. Supreme Court justices are appointed by the:

    A. President of the United States
    B. Congress
    C. Senate
    D. all of the above

14. A law that is prescribed by legislative enactments is known as:

    A. case law
    B. administrative law
    C. statutory law
    D. common law

15. Individuals are guaranteed certain fundamental freedoms by the Bill of Rights, including:

    A. freedom of speech
    B. equal protection
    C. due process
    D. all of the above

Matching

    A. felony

    B. common law

    C. criminal law

    D. statutory law

    E. misdemeanors

_____ 1. Also known as legislative law

_____ 2. Originally was developed in England

_____ **3.** Lesser crimes usually punishable by fines and imprisonment of less than 1 year

_____ **4.** Punishable by much larger fines and imprisonment for more than 1 year, or death

_____ **5.** Concerned with violations against society

Fill in the Blank

1. Crimes punishable by a fine or imprisonment for less than 1 year are called _____.

2. The execution of an unlawful or improper act is known as _____.

3. HIPAA is legislation that protects the consumer's right to _____.

4. Legislative law is also called _____.

5. Administrative law focuses on the regulation set forth and enforced by governmental administrative _____.

6. Rape and murder are examples of _____.

7. "Tort" is an Anglo-French word meaning _____.

8. The top court in a state may be called the _____.

9. Assault and battery or false imprisonment is an example of a/an _____.

10. The prescribing of medications by a person who isn't licensed describes the form of liability called _____.

CASE STUDY

The mother of a seven-month-old prematurely born infant was given a prescription for phenobarbital, which she took to her local pharmacist. A pharmacy technician, who did not have appropriate training and education to be a pharmacy technician, dispensed a strong oral expectorant medication instead of phenobarbital. Because the pharmacist was so busy, he decided not to check the medication or consult with the mother. She gave the medication to her child for about 1 month to prevent seizures. Because of the incorrect medication, the infant had a serious brain injury that caused a permanent disability.

1. Who is mostly responsible for this medication error?

2. What would be the consequences of severe seizures in this premature infant?

3. If a lawsuit claiming malpractice results, who may lose their jobs?

RELATED INTERNET SITES

http://biotech.law.lsu.edu

http://legal-dictionary.thefreedictionary.com

http://www.aspl.org

http://www.druglibrary.org; click on "Schaffer Library"

http://www.fda.gov; click on "Laws FDA enforces"

http://www.pharmacist.com; click on "pharmacy technicians"

http://www.rxtrek.net; click on "Enter RxTrek" and then "Certified Pharmacy *Technicians/Technologists (CPhT)*"; shows the number of certified pharmacy technicians across the U.S.

http://www.uscourts.gov/

REFERENCES

Abood, R. (2005). *Pharmacy Practice and the Law* (4th ed.). Jones and Bartlett.

Miller, R. D., & Hutton, R. C. (2000). *Problems in Health Care Law* (8th ed.). Aspen Publishers.

Reiss, B. S., & Hall, G. D. (2006). *Guide to Federal Pharmacy Law* (5th ed.). Apothecary Press.

CHAPTER 2

Ethics in Pharmacy Practice

OBJECTIVES

Upon completion of this chapter, the reader should be able to:

1. Define what is meant by the terms "legal" and "ethical."
2. Explain professional characteristics.
3. Define moral rights versus legal rights.
4. List three examples of how health care professionals may deal with mistakes.
5. Discuss the process used for making an ethical decision.
6. Explain why confidentiality is an ethical issue.

KEY TERMS

Autonomy – The ability or tendency to function independently.

Code of ethics – Standards developed to affect quality and ensure the highest ethical and professional behavior.

Ethics – The study of value, or morals and morality; it includes concepts such as right, wrong, good, evil, and responsibility.

Loyalty – A faithfulness or allegiance to a cause, ideal, custom, institution, or product.

Morals – Motivations based on ideas of right and wrong.

Professional ethics – Moral standards and principles of conduct guiding professionals in performing their functions.

Values – Desirable standards or qualities.

SETTING THE SCENE

A patient who is always very worried about her prescription medications arrives at the pharmacy with a prescription for metoprolol. The pharmacy technician knows this patient well and that she has high blood pressure, and often stops her medications because she is nervous about the side effects they sometimes cause. He fills her prescription and does not include the patient printout describing potential side effects and adverse reactions so that she will take the medication and not worry so much. The pharmacist instructs her on properly taking metoprolol and she leaves.

Critical Thinking

- What should the pharmacy technician have done to best benefit the patient in this situation?

- Is it legal for the technician to avoid including the patient printout that describes potential side effects and adverse reactions because he knows the patient well?

- Using the Internet, list five major adverse effects of metoprolol.

OVERVIEW

It is very important for pharmacy technicians to follow ethical standards of pharmacy practice, as well as exhibit professional behaviors that are of strong moral character. Technicians must always remember the value of the pharmacy profession, and how society and their own community trust in them.

Various pharmaceutical codes of ethics in the United States have been adopted and revised since 1848. The **code of ethics** established by the American Pharmaceutical Association was intended to publicly state the principles forming the fundamental basis of the roles and responsibilities of pharmacists. Likewise, the code of ethics for pharmacy technicians (as set forth by the American Association of Pharmacy Technicians) applies to pharmacy technicians working in any and all settings. This code of ethics is based on moral obligations that guide pharmacy professionals in relationships with their patients, other health-care professionals, and society in general.

ETHICS, MORALS, AND VALUES

Ethics are defined as *sets of principles of good conduct*, and also as *systems of moral values*. People commonly adopt ethics as part of a formal system of rules. **Morals** are defined as good principles or rules of conduct. They are more important socially than values. **Values** are desirable standards or qualities. They may also be defined as rules about right and wrong. Together ethics, morals, and values provide for rules of behavior upon which good character standards are established.

You Be the Judge

Phil is a pharmacy technician who is asked by a customer about Plan B®, which is intended for use as a morning-after pill. Because Phil believes that the use of a morning-after medication to prevent conception is wrong, he describes all sorts of serious adverse effects and states that they happen to most of the people who take the drug. As a result, the patient calls her doctor, who later calls the pharmacy and speaks with the pharmacist, telling him what Phil said and asking for an explanation. In your judgment, was Phil ethically correct in his actions? What sorts of legal repercussions do you think could await Phil as a result of his misstatements about Plan B?

Focus On...

Ethics

Ethics are standards of behavior developed as a result of society's concept of right and wrong.

Focus On...

Moral Values

Moral values consist of one's personal concept of right and wrong, formed through the influence of family, culture, and society.

THE RELATIONSHIP BETWEEN ETHICS AND THE LAW

In comparing ethics and law, it is important to understand the purposes, standards, and penalties that relate to each. Law is designed to protect society and help it to function efficiently by imposing civil or criminal penalties if laws are violated. In medicine, the law is designed to protect the rights of all individuals, be they patients, practitioners, or employees. Law enforcement may include fines, imprisonment, or sometimes both. Ethics are designed to assure adherence to standards while also serving to raise competence levels to build values. In the United States, the Medicare system was established with the intention of providing fair and ethical medical treatment for the elderly and the disabled. Ethical penalties include suspension from medical societies, decided by one's own medical peers.

PROFESSIONAL ETHICS

The term "professional ethics" is used only to denote "the profession's interpretation of the will of society for the conduct of the members of that profession augmented by the special knowledge that only the members of the profession possess." Professional ethics are concerned primarily with moral issues and responsibilities. Professionals must make informed decisions based on specialized training. They must act in the proper manner when their action is required to help or save the life of another. The medical profession and each of its separate areas have special codes of professional ethics that must be followed. The characteristics of a professional consist of a set of specific attitudes, which are essential for establishing professional ethics.

CODE OF ETHICS FOR PHARMACISTS

The American Pharmaceutical Association authored the Code of Ethics for Pharmacists. This code of ethics is based on moral obligations and designed to establish guidelines for professional ethical behavior. The central themes of the Code of Ethics for Pharmacists are:

- Pharmacists must respect the trust that their patients put upon them.

- They must always focus on the patient's well-being and comfort.

- The dignity and privacy of the patient must always be respected. Each patient's health is private information. The pharmacist should counsel patients so that they can make proper decisions about their own health.

- Pharmacists must always be truthful and non-discriminatory.

- They must continually keep aware of new advances in the field of pharmacy.

- The values of other professional colleagues must always be respected whenever they must be consulted.

- Though they focus on one patient at a time, the overall good of the community and society in general must always remain in their thoughts.

- Fair and equitable distribution of health resources must be maintained between patients and society.

Focus On...

Code of Ethics

A code of ethics for a health professional is a system of principles intended to govern behavior of those entrusted with providing care to the sick.

Visit the Web site of the American Pharmacists Association at http://www.pharmacist. com and search for "code of ethics" to find and review the Code of Ethics for Pharmacists.

The Patient-Pharmacist Relationship

The relationship between patients and pharmacists is one of the most critical in the medical field. A pharmacist must keep complete records on each patient in order to avoid medication errors or interactions that may result in harm. Some of the information that the pharmacist must manage includes lists of all medications that a patient is taking, including prescription, non-prescription, and herbal medications. It is important that the pharmacist establish a trusting relationship wherein the patient feels completely comfortable in discussing his or her health concerns with the pharmacist. The patient's complete medical history is vital in helping the pharmacist to understand his or her overall health picture, and to determine if any previous health issues may be related to his or her current condition. A patient's allergies are one of the most critical points of discussion, and patients must be instructed just how important their allergy information is in determining the correct medications to take. Any previous problems with medications should be noted, including unexpected reactions. Patients must be able to tell their pharmacist about previous, current, or planned pregnancies. They must be honest about their use of alcohol, tobacco, and recreational drugs if their health is to be maintained. These substances can and do interact with many different medications, and it is the continued job of the pharmacist to educate patients about how important the sharing of this information is.

Any time a pharmacist dispenses a new medication, be it to an existing patient or a new one, the patient should be counseled about the medication's effects. If anything is changed concerning the use of a medication (including dose, route of administration, and strength), the pharmacist and patient should communicate. The pharmacist must place patient counseling high on his or her priority list. Effective counseling establishes the solid patient-pharmacist relationship that can avoid misunderstandings that lead to medication errors. Strong effective communication between the patient and pharmacist helps to achieve the optimum outcome in treatment and care.

Patient Advocacy

Many health-care providers are required to represent patients while helping them to obtain health-care services and information. These patient advocates (health-care providers and pharmacists concerned with the cause and best interest of their patients) can assist in many different areas, including the choice of health care, getting needed information in order to make good health-care decisions, addressing how treatment will affect livelihood, discussing treatment with family members of the patient, watching for adverse effects, determining insurance coverage, and investigating alternative forms of treatment. Patient advocates can encourage patients to explain their symptoms fully in order to receive the best possible treatment. Most importantly, patient advocates must remember that the patient's health and well-being must remain the focus of their work.

Respect for Patient Autonomy

Autonomy is the ability or tendency to function independently. Patients must be allowed to decide their own medical care without being unduly influenced by health-care providers. Health-care providers must give the patient proper information in order to make an informed decision, but cannot actually decide for the patient. *Informed consent* is the term used to describe the patient's decision making related to his or her own health – it must be done after proper information has been given to the patient. Informed consent requires a patient to be competent to make decisions about his or her health. The decisions must be voluntary, using recommended strategies from qualified health-care providers. Patients must fully understand all of their options, and have had all information about their condition disclosed to them before deciding. Once the patient's decision has been made, he or she must give authorization to his or her health-care providers to proceed with whatever treatments the patient has decided upon. The American health-care system is fundamentally based upon ensuring the rights of patients.

> **What Would You Do?**
>
> It is a busy afternoon, and the pharmacy has only one pharmacy technician on duty. The pharmacist does not consult with two patients because of all his other responsibilities, and they leave the pharmacy. If you were the pharmacist in this situation, what should you have done?

Professional Competence

Professional competence is achieved over time, with continued learning and development. It is important to seek out continuing education and keep abreast of new technologies, developments, and the latest medical publications. Competency-based education has increased in popularity in the medical community, measuring student competence with specialized testing. This testing includes written exams, reviews by peers, and even self-assessment. Continuing education credits are required every few years. The goals of increased competence are focused on delivering the best health care possible to protect the public from disease.

Good communication skills, the ability to share information clearly and accurately, and the ability to keep information confidential are all required. Having an understanding of and empathy for others are important elements for quality pharmacy practice. Technical skills are also vital. These may include:

- Computer literacy
- Proficiency in English, science, and mathematics
- A willingness to learn new skills and techniques
- An ability to document well

Respect for Other Colleagues

It is important to always treat colleagues with respect. Discrimination results in no positive results, especially with colleagues alongside whom the pharmacist works on a regular basis. However, it is wise to challenge colleagues when they behave in less-than-professional ways. Criticism of their work should always be kept aboveboard – and never be unfair or cruel. Respect for other colleagues may be shown by being honest, on time, trustworthy, and a team player. Any unethical behavior shows a lack of respect for other colleagues, as it reflects on the workplace as a whole and may tarnish their reputations as well as that of the pharmacist.

Focus On...

Behavior

Unacceptable behaviors include theft, rudeness, lying, blaming, laziness, and complaining.

Serving the Community

Pharmacists are respected professionals on whom both patients and physicians rely. They are key allied health professionals who are trusted to provide safe and appropriate medications to the public. They serve their community by educating patients and consulting with them to prevent medication errors. Today, technology has changed greatly, and the role of pharmacists is more important than ever before.

Equitable Treatment

Pharmacists must always be ethical and moral. They cannot discriminate against patients for any reason (race, religion, color, financial status, etc.) and they must provide fair and equitable treatment. They must always follow their code of ethics to treat patients equally.

CODE OF ETHICS FOR PHARMACY TECHNICIANS

Pharmacy technicians, similar to pharmacists, should strive to make the care of every patient their utmost concern. They should always treat patients respectfully, responsibly, and honestly. Pharmacy technicians should use their best professional judgment at all times, and ask their pharmacist for advice if unsure about anything that occurs. They should encourage patients to speak directly with the pharmacist about any concerns. Professional competence must be continually maintained so that they can deliver the best health-care service.

The American Association of Pharmacy Technicians (AAPT) drafted its own version of a code of ethics distinct from that of pharmacists. Discussion of the central themes of the code of ethics for pharmacy technicians follows.

Focus On...

Pharmacy Technician's Code of Ethics

Search the Internet for the code of ethics for pharmacy technicians. Review this document. Print it and keep it on hand to periodically review.

Maintain Health and Safety

Pharmacy technicians are responsible for maintaining their own health so that they can be well enough to serve both pharmacists and customers. When a technician is physically or mentally ill, his or her health can interfere with the ability to provide good care to patients, or to safely execute professional pharmacy activities or decision-making. Pharmacy technicians must be cautious and careful in the practice of pharmacy. They must strive to avoid exposure to chemical substances in order to maintain both health and safety. In the workplace, safety is of the utmost importance to keep in mind. Maintaining good health for themselves and others is essential. To do this, all OSHA requirements must be met and followed (see Chapter 7).

You Be the Judge

Molly, a young pharmacy technician, goes into work early Monday morning after spending Sunday night out late at a nightclub with her friends. She has a bad hangover. How could Molly's condition affect her ability to provide good patient care? What could Molly have done instead of coming to work in this condition? What may be the consequences of this type of behavior?

Honesty and Integrity

Pharmacy technicians must always be honest, even when mistakes occur. Errors should be reported to supervisors immediately. All topics must be discussed factually, without exaggerations or distortions. The patient deserves to know the "straight truth," even if it is difficult to hear. Patient dignity is of utmost importance, and it can only be preserved by honesty and integrity in communications with them.

What Would You Do?

Sheila, a pharmacy technician, dropped a few capsules on the pharmacy floor while dispensing medications. Nobody else saw this happen. Quickly, she picked the capsules off the floor and put them back onto the tray, after which she included them in the container of dispensed medication. If you were Sheila, what would you do in this situation? If you were another pharmacy worker who saw this happen, what would you do?

Focus On...

Errors

Taking responsibility for your errors shows true integrity and character, and allows the mistake to be corrected.

Assist and Support the Pharmacist

The pharmacy technician assists the pharmacist with all tasks that they are allowed to perform by state law. The pharmacist must be supported in all activities so that he or she may perform his or her duties without distraction. The combination of a qualified and professional pharmacy technician with an equally competent pharmacist provides accurate and ethical health care that is as free of errors as possible. It is vital that the pharmacy technician supports the pharmacist's activities and adheres to instructions, bearing in mind all legal and ethical matters.

Respect for Other Health-Care Professionals

Staff members must work together for the good of their patients. Pharmacy technicians must be willing to perform duties outside of their formal job descriptions when they are needed to help in other areas of the pharmacy. Technicians must respect other health-care professionals and work as a team with them. Verbal and nonverbal communication is an important part in the establishment of respect for other health-care professionals. Ideally, everyone on the team should enjoy the workplace and get along with everyone else. This may be accomplished partially by setting aside personal feelings while at work, and cooperating with each other so that the job is performed efficiently.

Focus On...

Respect

You must treat each person, whether patient or coworker, the way you wish to be treated.

Professional Competence

Pharmacy technicians are under the direct supervision of pharmacists. The pharmacist is ultimately liable for the actions of the pharmacy technician, so extremely rigorous levels of competence are required. Pharmacy technicians must be able to balance busy daily activities with a strict adherence to detail. They must triple-check every drug that they dispense, all labeling, and the instructions provided by the physician as well as the pharmacist. As their job description evolves, pharmacy technicians are responsible for more duties than ever before, some of which used to be the sole responsibility of a licensed pharmacist. It is important that they alert the pharmacist to any discrepancies in information. The competence of a pharmacy technician is vitally important in today's pharmacy, and incompetent actions may result in legal action against the technician, the pharmacist, and the company they work for.

Respect for Patient Autonomy

Pharmacy technicians must have the ability to function independently. They must always show courtesy to patients in the pharmacy setting. A patient's freedom of choice, action, and thought is not to be interfered with. The pharmacy staff must respect self-governance, privacy, and patient choice. Kind words and compassion go far in building trust between technicians and patients. All pharmacy staff members should show kindness and consideration. The fact that someone is having a bad day does not excuse a display of anger or irritation with patients or other staff. A good attitude should be demonstrated consistently, and patients and visitors should be greeted with a smile.

Maintaining Confidentiality

Confidentiality is important in maintaining a patient's private information so that it does not become accessible to anyone who should not have access to it. Sharing private information with anyone who is not supposed to know it is a breach of ethics and may have legal ramifications. Those who do not respect and maintain confidentiality may be fired. Patient information, be it written, computerized, or even verbal, is not to be shared with anyone except approved health-care professionals. The Health Insurance Portability and Accountability Act (HIPAA) governs the disclosure of confidential information. Patients are usually required to read and sign a document that addresses to whom and under what circumstances their private medical information may be shared (see Chapter 5).

Observing Quality and Legal Standards

Pharmacy technicians must have knowledge of many techniques and principles, including related legal and ethical issues. Ethical standards are usually more severe and demanding than the standards required by law. Pharmacy technicians must also acquire a working knowledge of, and tolerance for, human nature and its individual characteristics. Daily contact with a wide variety of individuals with different problems and concerns is an important part of a pharmacy technician's duties. Courtesy, compassion, and common sense are vital to the success of the pharmacy technician.

Focus On...

Standards

A violation of either a legal or ethical standard can mean the loss of a technician's reputation.

Maintenance of Professional Standards

The pharmacy technician who works to improve his or her professional approach in the workplace will be a great asset to an employer. This ability will help them to be promoted to positions of more responsibility more quickly within the pharmacy. Therefore, maintenance of professional standards is essential for pharmacy technicians.

Loyalty to the Employer

Loyalty is defined as a faithfulness or allegiance to a cause, ideal, custom, institution, or product. Pharmacy technicians must appreciate the opportunity provided by their jobs in the pharmacy. They should support their workplaces by giving the best effort that they can. Today, many employees are interested in only what the employer can provide for them. This is an immature way to approach a job. When a technician is employed by a pharmacy, use of skills is exchanged for different types of compensation, with each benefitting the other. Often, pharmacy technicians forget that experience alone is a great benefit that they get from work. Supporting the employer with loyalty is important. Likewise, the pharmacy should loyally support its employees, including its pharmacy technicians.

The relationship between pharmacists and pharmacy technicians must be one of mutual respect and professionalism. Pharmacists have the ultimate responsibility over all of the actions of their pharmacy technicians. Clear communication between them is essential because any errors or negligence committed by the pharmacy technician will ultimately have to be answered for by the pharmacist. The pharmacist must check the accuracy of all of the pharmacy technician's actions.

What Would You Do?

Mr. Johnson, who has been coming to your pharmacy for many years, approaches you. You know that his wife died the previous year, and that he is taking medications to treat depression as well as cancer. When he arrives with a new prescription, he asks about the prescribed medication and comments, "I sure wouldn't want to take too much of this stuff. How much of this do you think would kill me if I wasn't careful?" Do you think Mr. Johnson may be contemplating suicide? What should you do first in this situation?

MAKING ETHICAL DECISIONS

A pharmacy technician must have a strong knowledge of ethical issues that might relate to their profession. They also must balance their own value systems with those of their profession.

An individual's life experience and values come into play when making good ethical decisions, which will occur on a daily basis. The effects their decisions can have on other individuals must be considered. Both long-term and short-term consequences must be taken into account.

Focus On...

Ethical Decisions

The responsibility for making a decision ultimately rests on the individual.

Identifying the Problem

Pharmacy technicians must focus on the individual problem that has occurred before making an ethical decision. They must think about various problems, both ethical and non-ethical, that may arise in the pharmacy. A pattern of behaviors must be established that will follow the identification of the problem.

Gathering Data

To gather information or data, pharmacy technicians should ask questions, review documentation, talk to patients and health-care professionals, and search for further data so that a complete picture of the situation becomes available. Once data is gathered, it can be scrutinized carefully. Then, an ethical problem can be identified correctly.

Analyzing the Data

After gathering data, the correct ethical approach in dealing with the situation must be decided upon. All individuals that are involved must be considered. This includes the consideration of their rights, job duties, and even personal character. Close attention should be paid to ramifications of all possible decisions, with alternatives considered and analyzed before action is taken.

Forming an Action Plan

When all the information about a situation has been gathered, the technician must then act properly and ethically. The action plan should begin to solve the problem. An action plan helps to evaluate all of the data and ascertain the various tasks that must be completed in order to handle a given situation. The good of a pharmacy's employees and patients results from situations that are handled properly, with fairness and forethought.

Evaluating the Results

After all steps have been taken to handle a problem or situation, it is important to evaluate the results that have occurred. Positive results that are fair and equitable to all are always desired. Proper evaluation of results helps to shape the way in which future decisions and problems will be solved in the pharmacy, with the ultimate result (good patient care and an effective staff) achieved.

ETHICAL ISSUES IN THE PHARMACEUTICAL INDUSTRY

It is important to understand that the interests of those who work in the pharmaceutical industry sometimes conflict or overlap with the interests of other health-care professionals. The exchange of gifts or money exemplifies serious ethical issues. As in every other area of this chapter, the patient's welfare must be placed above any other consideration. The costs of drug research and development are very large, and drug manufacturers must be able to recoup the money they spend. Sometimes, this can lead to unethical exchanges of medical or pharmacy practices for monetary or other entitlements. Legitimate patient care must be the goal of all medication development and manufacture, not monetary gain that leads to ethical breaches. Ideally, all forms of gifts should not be accepted by either pharmacy staff or physicians, but it is only through strong disciplinary or legal action that ethical or legal misappropriations may be ceased.

SUMMARY

Ethics exemplify principles of good conduct and moral behavior. Professional ethics are in place to ensure a level of quality of care and competence. They also serve to set a standard for professional behavior when dealing with patients and other colleagues.

The relationship between patients and pharmacists is one of the most critical in the medical field. Patients must be allowed to decide their own medical care without being unduly influenced by health-care providers, with their autonomy being respected. Likewise, respect for competent professional colleagues is important, with ethical and moral behavior being critical.

Pharmacists and pharmacy technicians must always be honest, even when mistakes occur. Errors should be reported immediately. Patient confidentiality must be maintained to ensure that private health information does not become accessible to anyone who is not authorized to have access to it. The patient's welfare must always be placed above any other consideration.

SETTING THE SCENE

The following discussion and responses relate to the opening "Setting the Scene" scenario:

- The pharmacy technician should have included the patient printout so that she would be able to read about the potential side effects and be less nervous about taking the medication. It would also be good to have reminded the pharmacist of the patient's history before patient counseling could occur.

- No, all dispensed prescriptions are required by law to include a patient printout that describes potential side effects and adverse reactions. The pharmacy technician should have included this regardless of his familiarity with the patient.

- Five major adverse effects of metoprolol include: agranulocytosis, hypoglycemia, bronchospasm, mental depression, and drowsiness.

REVIEW QUESTIONS

Multiple Choice

1. The Code of Ethics for Pharmacy Technicians is built upon which of the following perceived obligations?

   A. legal
   B. professional
   C. occupational
   D. moral

2. One of the characteristics of a professional is a set of specific:

   A. knowledge
   B. attitudes
   C. behaviors
   D. all of the above

3. One of the main considerations of the Code of Ethics for Pharmacy Technicians is to ensure the:

    A. patient's ability to economically afford medications
    B. prevention of dying and the health of the patient
    C. prevention of communicable diseases and safety
    D. health and safety of the patient

4. Morals are recognized as principles of:

    A. life and death
    B. an action or product
    C. faith
    D. right conduct

5. The American health-care system seems fundamentally based upon ensuring the:

    A. rights of patients
    B. coverage of prescriptions by insurance
    C. quantity of medications
    D. quality of pharmacy technicians

6. Lack of attention to detail or preoccupation with other activities may contribute to which of the following?

    A. conflicts of interest
    B. professional ethics
    C. confidentiality and fraud
    D. mistakes and errors

7. A student pharmacy technician asks a pharmacist (his uncle), "Why did my advisor recommend an ethics class for me?" Which of the following is the best response by the pharmacist?

    A. "Ethics must be learned in order to obey the law."
    B. "You may find studying ethics interesting."
    C. "It is the responsibility of pharmacy technicians to recognize ethical dilemmas in the workplace."
    D. "You must have misunderstood because pharmacy technicians do not have to study ethics."

8. Which of the following organizations approved the Code of Ethics for Pharmacy Technicians?

    A. the NAPT
    B. the AMA
    C. the APA
    D. the AAPT

9. A patient's self-governance, privacy, and right to liberty is described as:

   A. maintaining confidentiality
   B. professional competence
   C. patient autonomy
   D. legal standards

10. The patient's complete medical history is important in assisting the pharmacist to understand and determine:

    A. his or her previous health issues
    B. his or her overall health picture
    C. his or her allergy information
    D. all of the above

11. The pharmacist's actions of supporting and pushing for improvements in patient health-care issues is referred to as:

    A. patient advocacy
    B. patient confidentiality
    C. quality of medications
    D. professional competence

12. The profession's interpretation of the will of society that the conduct of the members of the profession display is referred to as:

    A. professional network
    B. professional ethics
    C. professional organization
    D. professional liability

13. The exchange of gifts or money exemplifies serious:

    A. professional issues
    B. pharmaceutical issues
    C. medical issues
    D. ethical issues

14. Technical skills for good communication include all of the following, except:

    A. proficiency in English, mathematics, and science
    B. practicing good sterile technique
    C. an ability to document well
    D. computer literacy

15. Motivations based on ideas of right and wrong are called:

    A. duties
    B. action plans
    C. morals
    D. needs

Fill in the Blank

1. The characteristics of a professional consist of a set of specific _____.

2. Each patient's health is _____ information.

3. The pharmacist must place patient counseling high on his or her _____ list.

4. The ability to function independently is called _____.

5. Pharmacy technicians must _____ check every drug that they dispense.

6. A good attitude should be demonstrated _____, and patients and customers should be greeted with a _____.

7. A pharmacy technician must have a strong knowledge of ethical issues that might relate to his or her _____.

8. The goals of increased competence are focused on delivering the best health care possible to protect the public from _____.

9. The Code of Ethics for Pharmacists was established by the American _____.

10. Professional competence must be continually maintained so that health-care professionals can deliver the best _____ services.

CASE STUDY

A celebrity who is spending time in the United States asks his doctor back home in England to prescribe some painkillers and antidepressants. The doctor complies according to the standards of his country, and the celebrity goes to a pharmacy in the United States to have the prescriptions filled. Because the pharmacy technician recognizes the celebrity, he begins dispensing the prescriptions. Meanwhile, the pharmacist also recognizes the celebrity, and begins to talk to him, asking what he is doing in the United States. He notices that the prescriptions originated in England, not the U.S.

1. What is the pharmacist's first responsibility regarding filling these foreign prescriptions?

2. Do you think that the pharmacist and pharmacy technician can fill these prescriptions under any circumstances?

3. Assuming that the celebrity received these prescriptions, and took them to commit suicide, who would be responsible for his death?

RELATED INTERNET SITES

http://changingminds.org; **click on "values" under the explanations section**

http://www.cancer.org; **search for "patient advocate"**

http://www.medterms.com

http://www.mja.com.au; **search for "ethics"**

http://www.op.nysed.gov; **search for "pharmacy"**

http://www.pharmacist.com; **search for "code of ethics for pharmacists"**

http://pharmpt.us.associationcareernetwork.com; **has information on job searches for pharmacy technicians**

REFERENCES

Burkhardt, M. A., & Nathaniel, A. K. (2008). *Ethics and Issues in Contemporary Nursing* (3rd ed.). Delmar, Cengage Learning.

Gauwitz, D. F. (2007). *Legal and Ethical Nursing.* Thomson/Delmar Learning.

Harris, D. M. (2003). *Contemporary Issues in Healthcare Law and Ethics* (2nd ed.). AUPHA/Health Administration Press.

Strandberg, K. M. (2002). *Essentials of Law and Ethics for Pharmacy Technicians.* CRC Press.

FEDERAL LAWS

Federal Regulation of Drug Products

OUTLINE

OBJECTIVES

Upon completion of this chapter, the reader should be able to:

1. Describe the purpose of the Pure Food and Drug Act.
2. Identify the reason that Congress adopted the Harrison Narcotics Tax Act.
3. Briefly explain the sulfanilamide tragedy.
4. Identify the concept of the Durham-Humphrey Amendment.
5. Explain the thalidomide tragedy.
6. Describe the purpose of the Kefauver-Harris Amendment.
7. Define OBRA-90 and explain the basic framework of it.
8. Describe the purpose of OSHA.
9. Explain the Drug Regulation Reform Act.
10. Describe the codes of the Drug Listing Act.

KEY TERMS

Adulteration – Tampering with or contaminating a product or substance.

Fraud – The intentional use of deceit to deprive another person of his or her money, property, or rights.

Fraudulent – Deceitful; intending to deceive.

Investigational – Drugs used to provide detailed inquiry or systematic examination of their effects.

Legend drug – Prescription drug.

Misbranding – Fraudulent or misleading labeling or marking.

National Drug Code (NDC) – The federal code that identifies a drug's manufacturer or distributor, its formulation, and the size and type of its packaging.

Orphan drug – Drugs used to treat diseases that affect fewer than 200,000 people in the United States.

Over-the-counter (OTC) – Non-prescription drug.

Phocomelia – A severe birth defect also known as "seal limbs," involving the malformation or non-formation of arms and legs; it was caused by the drug thalidomide.

Teratogenic – Causing genetic defects.

SETTING THE SCENE

A pharmacy technician dispensed a prescription in a non-child-resistant container. Her supervisor checked the medication and approved it. The patient left the pharmacy, only to return 3 days later. His grandson had opened the container and taken 15 pills. His physician had told him that this situation was the fault of the pharmacy.

Critical Thinking

- What did the pharmacy technician do wrong?
- What law was ignored? Explain this law.
- Who is responsible for this error and what may the consequences be?

OVERVIEW

The federal government enacts and interprets laws for the general population. State and local governments are responsible for determining the specifics of certain laws within their jurisdictions.

Regulatory agencies are government-based departments that create specific rules about what is and is not legal within a specific field or area of expertise. The regulatory agencies for the practice of pharmacy are the individual state boards of pharmacy. The U.S. Food and Drug Administration (FDA), which is a branch of the U.S. Department of Health and Human Services, regulates all drugs with the exception of illegal drugs. All legislation pertaining to drug administration is initiated, implemented, and enforced by the FDA. The FDA is responsible for the approval of drugs, over-the-counter (OTC) and prescription drug labeling, and standards for drug manufacturing.

Many laws and amendments that have shaped the current Food, Drug, and Cosmetic Act were enacted over the past 100 years. In most cases, they represent attempts on the part of lawmakers to protect the American public.

PURE FOOD AND DRUG ACT OF 1906

The Pure Food and Drug Act of 1906 prohibited the inter-state distribution or sale of *adulterated* (made impure with other ingredients) and misbranded (improperly labeled) food and drugs.

Almost 30 years after its enactment it was found to be inadequate for the following reasons:

1. It did not include cosmetics.
2. It did not provide authority to ban unsafe drugs.
3. A manufacturer could make false statements about a drug or medications.
4. Labels were not required to identify the contents of medications.

In 1912, Congress addressed the false statement problem and included within the definition of misbranding false and/or fraudulent claims for the curative powers of drugs. The Sherley Amendment to the act, which Congress enacted during 1912, first regulated labeling.

What Led to the Legislation?

The Pure Food and Drug Act was initiated because many products, including meats, patented medicines, and substances that contained cocaine, were sold to an unsuspecting public with labels that did not adequately describe the contents and the safety in consuming them. Many public figures, including those in politics and literature, complained about unsanitary and hazardous conditions that existed in the packaging of foods and drugs. They were opposed by many manufacturers who thought the proposed legislation would destroy their livelihoods.

Key Points of the Legislation

This act prevented the manufacture, sale, or transportation of impure (due to additives), misbranded, poisonous, or harmful drugs, foods, liquors, and medicines. It also controlled the traffic of these substances.

HARRISON NARCOTICS TAX ACT OF 1914

The Harrison Narcotics Tax Act of 1914 was implemented to regulate and tax the distribution, importation, and production of opiates. These substances included opium or coca products (which were used to manufacture cocaine). At this time, the distribution, sale, and use of cocaine was still legal for both companies and individuals. It is ironic that use of opiates and cocaine actually increased following the implementation of this act.

What Led to the Legislation?

Throughout the 1800s, opiates and cocaine were mostly unregulated. Many people were addicted to these substances, with as many as 1 in 400 U.S. citizens being addicted to opium itself. As time went on, an increasing number of crimes were linked to the use of opiates and cocaine. Public opinion began to sway toward prohibition – to ban alcohol and drugs.

Key Points of the Legislation

The legislation was intended to control the commerce of these drugs. It required drug manufacturers, sellers, distributors, importers, compounders, and dispensers to register with the Internal Revenue Service (IRS). The use of opium and coca leaves would be closely monitored from then on, and only for limited medical and scientific purposes. The term "narcotics" was used in the act's title to encompass both opiates as well as cocaine – though cocaine is not actually a narcotic (it is a central nervous system stimulant).

SULFANILAMIDE TRAGEDY OF 1937

In 1937, the Massengill Company introduced Elixir Sulfanilamide into the market. The elixir contained a solution with diethylene glycol. Sulfanilamide was a "sulfa" drug used to treat hemolytic streptococcal infections. Toxicity tests of the product were not conducted, and very little was known about the inherent toxicity of diethylene glycol (a deadly poison – now used as a type of permanent antifreeze used in automobiles). More than 100 patients died from ingesting Elixir Sulfanilamide before the FDA removed it from the market under a technical labeling violation of the 1906 Act; this became known as the sulfanilamide tragedy of 1937.

FOOD, DRUG, AND COSMETIC ACT OF 1938

The 1937 sulfanilamide tragedy propelled the passage of the Federal Food, Drug, and Cosmetic Act of 1938. Under this act, pharmaceutical manufacturers were required to file a New Drug Application with the FDA. Manufacturers had to ensure the purity, strength, safety, and packaging of drugs. Foods and cosmetics were also regulated. By this act, the FDA has the power to approve or deny new drug applications and even to conduct inspections to ensure compliance. The FDA approves the investigational use of drugs on humans and ensures that approved drugs are safe and effective.

This act remains the basis of today's law. The Food, Drug, and Cosmetic Act requires anyone who wishes to introduce a drug product to prove its safety to the FDA before it can be marketed. This Act was the beginning of the "pre-market approval process" for drugs in the United States, which requires the submission of a New Drug Application (NDA). For those interested, the entire Act may be found online at http://www.gpo.gov.

What Led to the Legislation?

The sulfanilamide tragedy of 1937 was of primary importance in the development of the Food, Drug, and Cosmetic Act of 1938. Because of the lack of testing, diethylene glycol was included in the Elixir Sulfanilamide and resulted in the mass poisonings.

Key Points of the Legislation

This act required drugs to be labeled with adequate directions so that they could be used safely. It also controlled cosmetic products and medical devices. It required all drugs to have FDA approval before they could be marketed. Manufacturers could not make false claims about the therapeutic properties of their medications. Standards of food packaging and quality could now be better enforced because of this act's requirements. Finally, it strengthened the FDA's ability to enforce the standards that it set forth.

DURHAM-HUMPHREY AMENDMENT OF 1951

During the 1940s, the FDA began to use internal regulations to create classifications of prescriptions (**legend drugs**), and non-prescription (**over-the-counter [OTC]**) drugs. This process did not work very well. Therefore, in 1951, Senator Hubert Humphrey, a pharmacist from Minnesota, and Congressman Carl Durham, a pharmacist from North Carolina, supported legislation to establish clear criteria for such decisions. The Durham-Humphrey Amendment of 1951 prohibits dispensing of legend drugs without a prescription. Non-legend OTC drugs were not restricted for sale and use under medical supervision.

This act created an exemption for drugs that could not be labeled safely for use by the public. Drugs marketed under this exemption could not be dispensed without prescriptions, but specific drugs were not indicated. A prescription that did not have refills indicated on its labeling when issued could still be refilled if the prescriber was contacted at a later date.

Focus On...

The Durham-Humphrey Amendment

The Durham-Humphrey Amendment allowed for verbal prescriptions over the phone and for refills to be called in from a physician's office.

What Led to the Legislation?

This legislation came about primarily because the FDA could not approve many important new drugs, such as antibiotics, under the existing law, because they could not be safely labeled without a physician's intervention. Before its establishment, many non-prescription and legend drugs bore little legal distinction regarding their use. Manufacturers regularly marketed directly to consumers without considering potential effects of the misuse of their products.

Key Points of the Legislation

This amendment required that drugs intended for use by humans that were not safe to use without medical supervision be dispensed only by prescription, and bear the legend "R_x." Drugs marketed as "by prescription only" were generally considered to be misbranded if dispensed without a prescription. This amendment required that legend drugs be labeled "Caution: Federal law prohibits dispensing without prescription." The use of the "R_x" symbol instead of this legend was the result of the later FDA Modernization Act (in 1997).

You Be the Judge

A pharmacy technician is working on a Saturday morning. His pharmacist decides to take a break since there are no customers in the pharmacy. During the pharmacist's break, a friend of the pharmacy technician enters the pharmacy and asks if he can have a few Percocet tablets because of back pain. The pharmacy technician gives his friend six Percocet tablets out of a container in the pharmacy. His friend takes these tablets and leaves. What do you think the pharmacy technician did wrong in this situation? If the pharmacist finds out about this, what do you think the consequences will be? What possible legal action could ensue against this pharmacy technician?

THALIDOMIDE TRAGEDY OF 1962

In 1961, the "thalidomide tragedy" began to unfold. Thalidomide was marketed in 1958 and was sold without prescription as a tranquilizer in West Germany until April 1961, when the drug was recognized as causing polyneuritis in adults. In November 1961, the drug was first believed to cause phocomelia (seal limbs), a severe birth defect. Thousands of infants had, by that time, been born in West Germany without one or both arms or legs, or with only partially formed limbs. The manufacturer withdrew the drug from the West German market on November 26, 1961.

Many drug firms had obtained licenses to market thalidomide on a worldwide basis. In the United States, the William S. Merrell Company had distributed the drug experimentally in 1960 under the trade name "Kevadon," but the FDA did not give final approval to the NDA that the company had submitted.

The FDA's timely action in withholding Kevadon approval was attributed to an FDA medical officer who refused approval while seeking data on further proof of safety. Even so, 29,413 patients in the United States had been involved in the human clinical trial testing of Kevadon. When the evidence that thalidomide was teratogenic (able to cause harm to a human fetus) was established, the FDA prevented the drug from reaching the market. As a result, only a small number of cases of phocomelia were reported in the United States. Thalidomide had been widely tested around the world as a tranquilizer, sedative, and as an anti-nauseant during pregnancy. Its widespread use for anti-nausea was what brought its detrimental adverse effects to the surface.

Focus On...

Thalidomide

The lesson of the thalidomide tragedy is that serious adverse effects can be caused by certain new drugs, as well as by new uses for older drugs. These adverse effects may not be discovered until very wide clinical use has occurred, as well as after some damage has taken place.

KEFAUVER-HARRIS AMENDMENT OF 1963

The Federal Food, Drug, and Cosmetic Act was amended again with the Kefauver-Harris Amendment of 1963 to require that drug products, both prescription and non-prescription, must be pure, effective, and safe. Prescription drug advertising was placed under supervision of the FDA and qualifications of drug investigators were subjected to review. These amendments provided for registration of manufacturers and inspection of manufacturing sites, and they required an unprecedented program of accountability from manufacturers.

What Led to the Legislation?

Senator Kefauver's ongoing study of trade practices within the drug industry, including the marketing of worthless and potentially dangerous drugs, led to the Kefauver-Harris Amendment. It was clear that the federal government needed further regulations in order to keep drug manufacturers from making worthless or dangerous drugs available to the public.

Key Points of the Legislation

This amendment required that all drug manufacturers prove the efficacy of the drugs to the FDA before they could be marketed. This meant that controlled studies had to be conducted which were thorough and rigorous. It specified that all drugs brought to market since the 1938 Food, Drug, and Cosmetic Act would have to meet the same requirements. Manufacturers had to report all adverse effects and also benefits to the FDA, and include such information in advertisements. Patients testing new drugs had to provide "informed consent," meaning that they had to be thoroughly educated about the possible medical risks of the drug they were testing.

COMPREHENSIVE DRUG ABUSE PREVENTION AND CONTROL ACT OF 1970

The Comprehensive Drug Abuse Prevention and Control Act of 1970 requires the pharmaceutical industry to maintain physical security and strict record keeping for many types of drugs. Its main achievement was to divide controlled substances into five categories called "schedules." Substances in Schedule I have the highest potential for abuse, while those in Schedule V have the least. Title II of this act is known as the Controlled Substances Act (CSA), and it is discussed in greater detail in Chapter 4. Drugs may be added or deleted from the schedules, as well as be changed to a different schedule, based on Drug Enforcement Agency (DEA) or Department of Health and Human Services (HHS) actions. Individuals and companies may also petition the DEA to add, delete, or change a drug's scheduling. The most important factor in placing a drug into a specific drug schedule is its potential for abuse. Any person who handles or intends to handle controlled substances must obtain a DEA registration. The DEA limits the amount of Schedule I and II substances that may be manufactured within the United States in a given 1-year period. Anyone manufacturing, distributing, or dispensing controlled substances in an unlawful manner is liable for prosecution under the rules of the CSA. A complete listing of drugs of abuse may be found at http://www.usdoj.gov (click on "DEA Home Page"; "Publications"; "Drugs of Abuse"; "Drugs of Abuse Chart").

What Led to the Legislation?

There were many laws and regulations in existence that dealt with dangerous drugs. Punishments for the use and sale of various substances were extremely wide-ranging, and not at all uniform. This led to confusion among the public and complicated the government's efforts in assuring compliance.

Key Points of the Legislation

This act was designed to update all previous laws that focused on the use and sale of narcotics and similarly dangerous substances. Possession of many substances was made illegal. The manufacturing and distribution of illegal drugs was given harsh penalties. The act also established standards to deal with drug abuse.

POISON PREVENTION PACKAGING ACT OF 1970

The Poison Prevention Packaging Act authorized the Consumer Product Safety Commission to create standards for child-resistant packaging. Its "special packaging" terminology signifies containers made to be very difficult for young children to open. This act requires that a few OTC drugs, and nearly all legend drugs, be packaged in child-resistant containers that cannot be opened by 80 percent of children younger than 5 years, but can be opened by 90 percent of adults (see Figure 3-1). It requires pharmacists

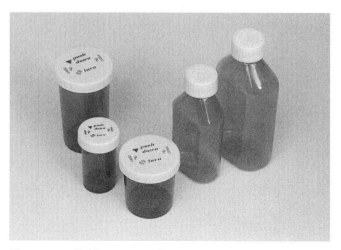

Figure 3-1 Child-resistant safety caps.

to dispense certain drugs in child-resistant containers. Drugs dispensed for use by patients in hospitals or nursing homes are usually not required to be packaged in child-resistant containers because children usually do not have access to them in these environments. However, assisted-living environments are considered "households," and child-resistant containers are usually required. Stock bottles of medications do not usually require special packaging because they are intended to be used by pharmacists for repackaging of drugs prior to dispensing. It is important that pharmacy technicians also understand that many "blister packs" (such as the Z-Pak) are considered child-resistant under the provisions of this act.

If a prescriber authorizes non-child-resistant containers, they may be provided by the pharmacist. Also, if a patient (for example, an elderly or handicapped patient) requests non-child-resistant containers, they may likewise be provided by the pharmacist. Non-child-resistant containers are commonly labeled "Package Not Child Resistant" or "This Package For Households Without Young Children." It is important that pharmacy personnel ascertain that there are no young children who might potentially come in contact with the medication containers prior to dispensing medications in non-child-resistant containers. A signed release form confirming the patient's request should be placed into the patient record. Legally, the patient must sign the back of the original prescription, requesting a non-child-resistant container. Pharmacy technicians should also check the box on the patient profile indicating his or her preference for non-child-resistant containers.

"Reminder" packaging (commonly referred to as "Bingo cards" or "Medisets") are not compliant with this act, so a request must be obtained from the patient in order to approve these non-child-resistant types of containers. Medications that do not need to be placed in a child-resistant container include the following, though these often have specific dosage requirements that apply:

- Betamethasone, prednisone, mebendazole, or methylprednisolone tablets
- Chewable isosorbide dinitrate
- Erythromycin ethylsuccinate granules, suspension, or tablets
- Potassium supplements
- Powdered anhydrous cholestyramine and colestipol
- Sodium fluoride or pancrelipase preparations
- Sublingual nitroglycerin or isosorbide dinitrate

Another method of avoiding potential poisonings is the use of tamper-resistant prescription pads. These are designed so that anyone using them fraudulently will be caught due to hidden components that they contain. They feature erasure protection to keep users from changing information by erasing what may have previously been written by an authorized prescriber; control batch numbers; and hidden watermarks.

What Led to the Legislation?

Many young children ingested poisonous or toxic substances before this act was established. Aspirin was the first substance that had to be packaged with childproof lids because of this act. Included under this act's legislation are corrosive, irritative, and toxic substances.

Key Points of the Legislation

The Poison Prevention Packaging Act requires that the types of substances referenced above be packaged in a way that makes it difficult for children younger than five years to open them. It provides that the same packaging should be easy for most adults to open. Regarding medications, nearly all prescription medications, with a few exceptions (such as nitroglycerin) must be packaged in this manner, and some OTC medications must be similarly packaged. Adult patients who may have trouble opening their medications (because of conditions such as arthritis) may decline to receive child-resistant packaging, though they must sign a release form to document their request.

OCCUPATIONAL SAFETY AND HEALTH ACT (OSHA) OF 1970

In 1970, Congress passed the Occupational Safety and Health Act to prevent workplace disease and injuries. This statute applies to virtually every U.S. employer. The general purpose of the act is to require all employers to ensure employee safety and health.

The Occupational Safety and Health Act includes regulations for physical workplaces, machinery and equipment, first aid, and job-related materials. It was intended to require employers to provide safe and healthy working conditions. It ensures that workplaces must be free of recognized hazards. These may include dangerous machinery, excessive noise, extreme temperatures, toxic chemicals, or unsanitary conditions. The Occupational Safety and Health Administration (also called OSHA) was established by this act. This administration is discussed in detail in Chapter 7.

What Led to the Legislation?

For many years, workers were at the mercy of their employers in regard to the safety and healthfulness of their work environments. Since the advent of mechanized production equipment, injuries at the workplace became more common. Until the development of this act, and the Occupational Safety and Health Administration, there was little government regulation concerning the safety and health of employees. After World War II, workplace-related deaths peaked at approximately 14,000 per year.

Key Points of the Legislation

OSHA was established to protect the health and safety of workers in the private sector as well as governmental jobs. Its key points are the protection of workers from chemicals, lack of sanitation, machinery, noise, and extreme temperatures. The act also created the Occupational Health and Safety Review Commission to ensure proper enforcement of its standards.

DRUG LISTING ACT OF 1972

Under the Drug Listing Act, each new drug is assigned a unique and permanent drug code. This code is known as a **National Drug Code (NDC)** that identifies the manufacturer or distributor, the drug formulation, and the size and type of its packaging. The FDA uses this code to maintain a database of drugs by use, manufacturer, and active ingredients, and of newly marketed, discontinued, and remarketed drugs. Each drug is assigned an 11-digit NDC number. The first five digits identify the manufacturer. The next four digits represent the drug product, and the last two digits determine the package size or type of packaging. An example of an NDC number is as follows: 00135-0315-52 (the first segment is the labeler code, assigned by the FDA; the second segment is the product code; and the third segment identifies the package size). Pharmacy technicians should understand that the accurate tracking of an NDC number is the key in avoiding audit problems regarding Medicaid or Medicare. If an insurance claim is filed using the wrong NDC, **fraud** charges against the person who filed the claim may result.

Focus On...

NDC

The NDC for a certain product may not be used for another if any changes occur in the product's characteristics. A new NDC number must be assigned to the new version of the product.

What Led to the Legislation?

Prior to this act, many drug products were misbranded or labeled incompletely or incorrectly. Drug data was often improperly reported to the FDA. Changes to drug products were often made without a new National Drug Code (NDC) number being applied for.

Key Points of the Legislation

This act amended the Food, Drug, and Cosmetic Act of 1938. It required all drug manufacturers to list all of their commercial products with the FDA. Its jurisdiction reaches from the manufacturer, through every individual or company that handles the drug product, up to the final point of sale. It requires that drug product listings be updated two times per year.

What Would You Do?

David is a pharmacy technician who received a prescription of Valium 50 mg b.i.d. for 30 days, with 5 refills. After thoroughly reviewing this prescription, if you were David, what would you do?

MEDICAL DEVICE AMENDMENT OF 1976

In 1976, medical devices previously subject to control only under the Food, Drug, and Cosmetic Acts general **adulteration** and misbranding sections were subjected to extensive new requirements. In order to keep up with rapidly expanding scientific and medical technology, devices were classified and subjected to different levels of control, depending upon how their function was evaluated. The safety and effectiveness of life-sustaining and life-supporting devices were required, for the first time, to have the pre-market approval of the FDA.

Focus On...

Medical Devices

Pharmacy technicians must be familiar with many medical devices in the pharmacy. Commonly used devices in the pharmacy include scales, pill-counting devices, wheelchairs, crutches, and others.

What Led to the Legislation?

Failures and problems surrounding pacemakers and intrauterine devices (IUDs) were among the chief influencing factors regarding this act. Prior to this legislation, the FDA had little ability to regulate medical devices for safety, effectiveness, and proper use.

Key Points of the Legislation

The Medical Device Amendment of 1976 classified medical devices according to their risk levels. It set up three different classes of devices. While Class I and II devices do not require pre-market approval, Class III devices have to pass unique regulatory requirements.

RESOURCE CONSERVATION AND RECOVERY ACT OF 1976

The Resource Conservation and Recovery Act of 1976 is also referred to as the Solid Waste Disposal Act. It regulates the handling of solid wastes and authorizes environmental agencies to handle the cleanup of contaminated sites. It also regulates solid waste landfills. It focuses on the protection of human, animal, and environmental health and welfare by reducing and eliminating pollution.

What Led to the Legislation?

This act was required because of large-scale disposal of hazardous wastes in ways that could lead to environmental pollution and poisonings of humans and animals. Before the Resource Conservation and Recovery Act, there was little forethought or planning completed prior to the dumping of hazardous waste.

Key Points of the Legislation

This act regulates the ways in which hazardous wastes must be disposed of. It gives environmental agencies the power to order approved methods of cleaning up improperly disposed wastes. It encouraged that open dumps or landfills be eliminated, and that comprehensive solid waste management programs be developed.

DRUG REGULATION REFORM ACT OF 1978 AND PROVISIONS

This act was intended to revise the Food, Drug, and Cosmetic Act on many different levels. It did not pass in 1978. In 1979, the Act was approved by the Senate. Ultimately however, the House did not act on its approval. The Drug Regulation Reform Act of 1978 contained nine provisions, as follows:

1. To increase consumer protection
2. To encourage drug innovation
3. To increase consumer information
4. To protect patient rights

5. To improve FDA enforcement

6. To promote competition and cost savings through generic drugs

7. To increase the FDA's public accountability

8. To make additional drugs available

9. To encourage research and training

What Led to the Legislation?

Lack of drug regulation and the need for fairer consumer protection prompted this revision of the Food, Drug, and Cosmetic Act. High drug prices, due to lack of competition in the industry, were also instrumental in its development.

Key Points of the Legislation

The Drug Regulation Reform Act and its provisions were designed to encourage fairer FDA regulation of the pharmaceutical industry. It was focused on shortening the time required to develop new drugs, get approval, and bring them to market. It was also intended to reduce the costs involved in the development of new drugs so that manufacturers would be able to develop more drug products at lower cost.

DRUG RECALLS

Manufacturers may determine that a drug they manufacture has been shown to be harmful to the public. When this occurs, they may issue a drug recall, and inform the FDA. Also, the FDA may recommend that a drug be recalled by its manufacturer. However, though the FDA can withdraw approval of a drug, products marketed prior to the withdrawal of approval may remain on the market. The FDA may obtain a warrant to seize defective products, but this is not a drug recall. The FDA can recall defective animal foods, medical devices, and infant formulas. Because the FDA can take legal action against a manufacturer of a harmful drug product, it is best that the manufacturer voluntarily announce the recall and inform the FDA. Serious injury and even death has resulted from several drugs on the market, and over a dozen drugs have been recalled or withdrawn in recent years. Some of these include:

- Avandia – it was withdrawn until a black box warning could be added because it has been shown to cause or worsen heart failure in some patients

- Ortho Evra birth control patch – the manufacturer was required to withdraw this product and update its warning label due to patients who experienced blood clots, deep vein thrombosis, heart attack, pulmonary embolisms, and stroke

- Vioxx – it was recalled due to thousands of lawsuits from patients and their families related to fatal arrhythmias and heart diseases

- Ceclor suspension – it was recalled because of drying agent (desiccant) packets that were found in some bottles, and the manufacturer feared potential adulteration of the product

Focus On...

Drug Recalls

The manufacturer may issue a drug recall on its own, or it may do so according to a request by the FDA.

There are three classes of drug recalls:
- *Class 1 – the most severe type of FDA recall, these occur when there is a serious potential for injury or death*
- *Class 2 – these occur when there is a less serious potential for injury or death, but still the possibility of serious adverse effects that may have consequences that are irreversible*
- *Class 3 – these occur where there is the potential of adverse effects even though they are not very likely*
- *Market withdrawal – a manufacturer's removal or correction of a distributed product which involves a minor violation that is not subject to legal action by the FDA, or no actual violation, but when the manufacturer decides to correct something about the product*

When a drug recall is issued, the pharmacy technician must assist the pharmacist in removing all of the drug product from the shelves, packaging the recalled drug product for return to the manufacturer, and contacting anyone who has received the drug product in question from the pharmacy so that they can be alerted about the recall. In these circumstances, they must follow all of the guidelines of the pharmacy concerning drug recalls, which should be listed in the pharmacy's policies and procedures manual.

ORPHAN DRUG ACT OF 1983

The Orphan Drug Act of 1983 offers federal financial incentives to commercial and nonprofit organizations for the development and marketing of drugs previously unavailable in the United States. Before a new drug can be marketed, substantial evidence of its safety and effectiveness must be proven. This procedure is difficult, lengthy, and extremely expensive. Previously, valuable new drugs with efficacy for a disease that affected only a small number of people were not being developed because manufacturers did not want to invest both the money and time needed to secure approval. A drug that falls into this category is called an **orphan drug**. These drugs are used to treat diseases affecting fewer than 200,000 people in the United States. This act offers tax breaks and a 7-year monopoly on drug sales in order to induce companies to undertake the development and manufacturing of such drugs. Since the Act went into effect in 1983, more than 100 orphan drugs have been approved. Orphan drugs include those used for the treatment of acquired immunodeficiency syndrome (AIDS), cystic fibrosis, blepharospasm (uncontrolled rapid blinking), and snakebites.

Focus On...

Orphan Drugs

The law provides exclusive licensing and tax incentives for manufacturers to develop and market orphan drugs.

What Led to the Legislation?

This act was established because of many different diseases and conditions that existed in the United States but affected 200,000 individuals or less. These diseases and conditions included ALS (aka "Lou Gehrig's Disease"), Huntington's disease, muscular dystrophy, myoclonus (abnormal muscle contraction), and Tourette's syndrome. Prior to this act, there were few medications that could treat these and other rare conditions.

Key Points of the Legislation

This act offered tax breaks and a 7-year monopoly to manufacturers of orphan drugs, and therefore helped to make the manufacture of these drugs profitable for their makers. It covered about 5,000 different rare conditions.

DRUG PRICE COMPETITION AND PATENT TERM RESTORATION ACT OF 1984

The Drug Price Competition and Patent Term Restoration Act of 1984 gave marketers of a generic drug the ability to file "abbreviated new drug applications" to seek FDA approval of the generic drug. This act was created to give more incentives to drug manufacturers in order to offset the time and money required to bring new, innovative drug products to market. In most cases, it allows previous patents to be extended by 5 years. Overall, this act has greatly helped in the generic drug approval process.

In the pharmacy, the "Orange Book" is used for the approval of drug products with therapeutic equivalence. This book evaluates these drug products to ensure safe substitutions. Now also in electronic format, the Orange Book allows searching by active ingredients, proprietary name, applicant holder, or applicant name. There are different versions of this book, with updates being available as frequently as every month.

What Led to the Legislation?

Drug manufacturers did not, prior to this act, have good patent protection for new drugs that they brought to market. They also did not have enough market exclusivity to ensure that their new drug products remained unique to them. Without a sufficiently long period of drug product exclusivity, manufacturers simply could not recoup their drug development costs.

Key Points of the Legislation

This act amended the Food, Drug, and Cosmetic Act. It created a formal generic drug approval process and established the abbreviated new drug application (ANDA) approval process. Under this act, generic versions of innovator drugs that had been approved earlier could get FDA approval without the manufacturer having to submit a full new drug application (NDA).

Focus On...

How a Drug Comes to Market

There are three clinical phases that must be completed before a drug is made available in the U.S. Phase 1 studies are designed to determine the drug's safety, adverse effects, and metabolism. Phase 2 studies target the drug's effects upon people with certain conditions or diseases. Phase 3 studies weigh the drug's safety and effectiveness compared to differing dosages, use with other drugs, and among different populations. The FDA reviews these studies and may require Phase 4 studies to study information about new populations, long-term effects, and new dosages. Phases 1, 2, and 3 commonly take from 2 to 10 years. Additionally, post-marketing surveillance occurs throughout the life of use of the drug product.

PRESCRIPTION DRUG MARKETING ACT OF 1987

The Prescription Drug Marketing Act of 1987 was enacted to ensure that prescription drug products are safe and effective, and to avoid tainting, counterfeiting, and misbranding of drugs. Its main purpose is to protect the ability of drug manufacturers to maintain different pricing to different segments of the market. It also allows for effective control over drug sources. This act regulates the methods of selling specific drugs and controls those companies and individuals who participate.

What Led to the Legislation?

The development of a "diversion market" (a wholesale submarket) of prescription drugs was the main factor in this act being passed. This sub-market consisted of many unauthorized distributors marketing prescription drugs to buyers who intended to use them for recreational use, and operating with little government intervention. Another influencing factor was that certain facilities that dealt with blood products were distributing blood-derived products with no regulation.

Key Points of the Legislation

This act established specific prescription drug distribution standards. It encouraged the distribution of authentic, properly labeled, and effective prescription drugs. It required that wholesalers of prescription drugs be state-licensed. It also regulated blood centers that provided certain health-care services and controlled their ability to distribute blood-derived products.

OMNIBUS BUDGET RECONCILIATION ACT OF 1990

The Omnibus Budget Reconciliation Act of 1990, also known as OBRA-90, contained important amendments affecting Medicare and Medicaid. Its main purpose was to reduce Medicaid costs by reducing inappropriate use of drugs by Medicaid recipients. Though there is currently no cap on Medicare taxes, this act created a tax limit cap on taxable income (as of 2008, this cap is $102,000). The act is administered by the Centers for Medicare and Medicaid Services. It requires Medicaid pharmacy providers to obtain, record, and maintain basic patient information, including disease history. Pharmacy technicians assist in the maintenance and updating of patient profiles.

OBRA-90 expanded rules about drug products to ensure the utmost safe and effective drug therapy, effectively prohibiting the prescription of legend drugs for unapproved uses. It helps patients to save money while obtaining the quality medications they need by offering rebates, scientific studies, and drug use review. OBRA-90 expanded on the act known as OBRA-87, which included the Nursing Home Reform Act of 1987. This act required monthly review of Medicare and Medicaid patients in nursing homes, and periodic reviews of psychotropic drug use in nursing homes. It was designed to provide the highest quality care for residents of nursing homes.

OBRA-90 also requires that each state must require its pharmacists to offer to counsel each of their patients (including Medicaid patients) and review the drugs they have been taking. Pharmacy technicians should ascertain that the pharmacist has counseled each and every patient. Medicaid demands that these procedures, as well as pharmacist maintenance of Medicaid patient profiles and the performance of prospective drug use reviews, are completed for each and every covered patient in order for funding to continue. Significantly, OBRA-90 requires that manufacturers provide the lowest prices to Medicaid patients by rebating each state Medicaid agency the difference between the average price and the lowest available price, though this does not directly help patients to save money. Each state is required to establish a board that reviews drug use in order to detect fraud or inappropriate care from physicians or pharmacists.

Focus On...

Drug Use Review

In order to make sure that drug therapy for patients is as safe and effective as it can be, OBRA-90 requires drug use evaluation (DUE). This process consists of analyzing a patient's medications to ensure that there is no duplication, as well as checking any and all contraindications, interactions, patient allergies, correct dosages, and proper term of usage.

What Led to the Legislation?

Prior to this act, many Medicaid patients received less than quality care, and experienced high medical costs. Lack of prospective drug use review, poor patient counseling, and bad maintenance or patient records also contributed to the establishment of this act.

Key Points of the Legislation

This act requires pharmacists to review Medicaid patients' complete drug profiles before filling their prescriptions. They must offer to discuss each patient's drug-therapy regimen with him or her. Certain basic information must now be included in each Medicaid patient's personal profile. State Medicaid programs must maintain a Drug Use Review Board.

FDA Safe Medical Devices Act of 1990

This act gives the FDA increased ability to regulate medical devices and products used for medical diagnosis. Also known as the SMDA, it requires medical device reports to be filed on a timely basis. It established an approval procedure for new medical devices prior to their becoming available on the market. The SMDA also increased civil penalties for anyone violating the Food, Drug, and Cosmetic Act's policy on medical devices.

What Led to the Legislation?

Prior to this act, medical devices had little regulation. When these devices caused patient harm or death, the injured parties had inadequate federal support for their cases.

Key Points of the Legislation

This act requires facilities that use medical devices to report the devices if illness, injury, or death occurs because of their use. It controls the method of reporting such devices and protects those that report them. It also requires better manufacturer quality control and tracking of the devices that they bring to market.

Anabolic Steroids Control Act of 1990

This act allowed the Controlled Substances Act to regulate anabolic steroids. These hormonal substances promote muscle growth, and are often used illegally by athletes. Also known as "performance-enhancing drugs," anabolic steroids have been shown to have serious health consequences from overuse. The Anabolic Steroids Control Act is considered significant because it sparked a new era of the control of drug abuse. This act offered harsher penalties for the abuse and misuse of anabolic steroids by athletes.

You Be the Judge

A pharmacy technician who is also an avid basketball player has begun using anabolic steroids, obtained illegally from the pharmacy in which he works. Slowly, his behavior begins to change as a result of these drugs, and he soon is fired from his job. What are the most common adverse effects of using anabolic steroids? Is the pharmacist liable for not noticing that these drugs were being taken? What would be the consequences of stealing anabolic steroids?

What Led to the Legislation?

Prior to this act, anabolic steroids were obtained and used with more ease, and with less regulation, than they are now. The abuse of anabolic steroids by athletes and others who were interested in increasing muscle growth led to serious consequences and even death.

Key Points of the Legislation

This act put anabolic steroids into Schedule III of the CSA. It raised penalties for illegal distribution of these agents, as well as for human growth hormone. It resulted in the prosecution of many foreign companies who were distributing these types of products into the U.S. market.

AMERICANS WITH DISABILITIES ACT OF 1990

This act prohibits discrimination against disabled persons. It focuses on areas that concern employment, public services and transportation, public accommodations and commercial facilities, telecommunications, and more. The Americans with Disabilities Act, also known as the ADA, oversees issues concerning devices and accommodations that disabled persons need in order to live as normally as possible, and their rights surrounding these devices and accommodations. Disabled persons cannot be subjected to medical examinations prior to employment that would not be given to all prospective employees.

Focus On...

ADA

This law prevents discrimination against potential employees who possess a disability.

What Led to the Legislation?

Companies that denied fair treatment to those with disabilities became the focus of many groups who were advocates for the disabled, hence the adoption of this act.

Key Points of the Legislation

This act prohibits discrimination against the disabled, regardless of whether their impairment is physical or mental. It provided clear standards of enforcement against those who discriminate against the disabled. It protects the civil rights of the disabled in a similar way to how previous civil rights legislation protected against discrimination concerning race, sex, religion, and other topics.

DIETARY SUPPLEMENT HEALTH AND EDUCATION ACT OF 1994

This act was intended to amend the Food, Drug, and Cosmetic Act. Its focus was to change the way in which dietary supplements are labeled and regulated. It is important to remember that dietary supplements have always been, and still are, treated as foods, not drugs. Also known as the DSHEA, this act holds dietary-supplement manufacturers responsible for the safety of the supplements they manufacture. The Dietary Supplement Health and Education Act of 1994 controls many types of dietary supplements, including amino acids, herbs and different types of botanicals, some hormones, minerals, vitamins, and other dietary supplements.

This act affects pharmacy technicians regarding the displaying, stocking, and recommendation of supplements. In the pharmacy, technicians are not allowed to recommend dietary supplements, just as they are not allowed to recommend OTC or legend drugs. Pharmacy technicians are, under this act, not allowed to attach extraneous labeling or stickers to the packages of dietary supplements.

What Led to the Legislation?

Before the Dietary Supplement Health and Education Act of 1994, various substances and formulations were sold as supplements with little or no regulation. This led to dangerous interactions with prescription and OTC drugs, and caused patient harm. It was clear that some sort of regulation was necessary for dietary supplements.

Key Points of the Legislation

This act clearly defined the term "dietary supplement." It enforced regulations against any manufacturer of a dietary supplement that claimed that the supplement actually treated or cured a specific condition.

HEALTH INSURANCE PORTABILITY AND ACCOUNTABILITY ACT (HIPAA) OF 1996

HIPAA was designed to improve continuity and portability of health insurance, to reduce fraudulent activities, to establish medical savings accounts, to improve long-term health-care access, and to simplify health-care administration. It also sought to improve the effectiveness of Medicare and Medicaid by improving the system used to store and share private health information. HIPAA provides for health-care coverage for workers who lose or change their jobs. It developed national provider identifiers (NPIs) for health-care providers, employers, and health insurance plans. A national provider identifier is a unique identification number for covered health-care providers. An NPI consists of 10 digits with no letters or other characters. These numbers are easy to obtain and are free. They are especially essential for providers who bill Medicare for services.

HIPAA regulations are divided into three parts: privacy regulations, security regulations, and transaction standards. The privacy regulations give patients specific rights, which include: access to their records, accounting of disclosures, hospital privacy, amendments to their records, communication of health information, and use/disclosure of information. The security regulations are designed to ensure the confidentiality of protected health information. The transaction standards require common code sets, common electronic claims standards, and unique health identifiers (see Chapter 5).

What Would You Do?

Mary Jo, an inexperienced pharmacy technician, started working in a retail pharmacy last week. Many customers were in close proximity to the counter. While dispensing a prescription for a certain patient, she called out to her by name, asking, "Mrs. Corby, can you please give me your Medicaid card so that I can make a copy?" What would you do in this situation, and what law was violated by Mary Jo?

What Led to the Legislation?

Prior to HIPAA, many employees who changed or lost their jobs could not maintain their health insurance coverage. There was a lack of cohesiveness in how standards concerning health care and insurance were administered. The health-care system needed some sort of constancy and better overall organization.

Key Points of the Legislation

HIPAA protects health insurance coverage after the loss or changing of a job. It established national standards for health-care transactions, and national identifiers for individuals and companies within the system. It encouraged electronic data interchange of private health information. For the pharmacy, HIPAA requires a signed notice that describes the protection of private health information.

FDA MODERNIZATION ACT OF 1997

This act was designed to reform the regulation of cosmetics, food, and medical products, focusing primarily on user fees, safe pharmacy compounding, food safety, and regulation of medical devices. It increased patient access to experimental drugs and medical devices. This act also passed incentives giving manufacturers 6-month extensions on new pediatric drugs that had drug trial testing data on file. Importantly, it also mandated risk assessment reviews of all foods and drugs that contain mercury in the United States. Also known as the FDAMA, this act changed the promotion of off-label drugs significantly. This law required that manufacturers of legend drugs must label their packaging with the "R_x" symbol.

Medicare Part D was established to subsidize prescription drug costs for Medicare beneficiaries. This drug benefit may be obtained by either joining a prescription drug plan (PDP) or a Medicare Advantage (MA) plan. Enrollment is voluntary and occurs annually. Plans can be tailored to cover different drugs, or classes of drugs, and various co-payment amounts. Medicare Part D does not cover drugs that are not approved by the FDA, those not intended for their approved indications, those not available for prescribing within the U.S., and those already covered by Medicare Parts A or B. Also excluded are drugs or drug classes excluded from Medicaid coverage.

What Led to the Legislation?

Prior to this act, the drug approval process was slow and rather cumbersome. This act was intended to speed up the process so that the benefits of new medications and therapies could be enjoyed by the public on a timely basis.

Key Points of the Legislation

This act was passed to improve FDA regulation of drugs, biological products, food, and medical devices, with the main aim of speeding up the approval process. It was poised to address the changing technologies and marketing of these products in relation to the growing, diversifying public.

MEDICARE PRESCRIPTION DRUG, IMPROVEMENT, AND MODERNIZATION ACT OF 2003

Also known as the Medicare Modernization Act (MMA), this act overhauled the Medicare program more than any other act. It introduced tax breaks and subsidies for prescription drugs. This act presents new Medicare "Advantage" plans that offered patients better choices about their terms of care, providers, other types of coverage, and federal reimbursements. Significantly, the MMA established a trial, partially privatized Medicare system, offered pretax medical savings accounts, and raised certain fees for wealthier senior citizens.

What Led to the Legislation?

Newer and more expensive drugs regularly came to market since 1965, when Medicare was created. Many patients, with senior citizens leading the way, found it hard to afford these new drugs. This act was established to help them.

Key Points of the Legislation

This act provided an entitlement benefit for prescription drugs. It used subsidies and tax breaks in order to help them afford the medications they needed. It also offered employers to offer drug benefits to their employees through drug subsidies.

ISOTRETINOIN (ACCUTANE®) SAFETY AND RISK MANAGEMENT ACT (PROPOSAL ONLY) OF 2005

This act was proposed, but not passed, to establish certain restrictions concerning drugs that contained isotretinoin (Accutane®). It was designed to restrict the distribution of Accutane and monitor the drug's side effects. The act was proposed because this drug, used to treat acne, can cause severe birth defects in the fetuses of patients who take Accutane during pregnancy. This drug has also caused spontaneous abortions to occur. Since this act failed to be passed, the FDA has initiated a program known as "SMART" (System to Manage Accutane Related Teratogenicity). However, the SMART program has not significantly reduced cases of Accutane-related birth defects and fetal deaths.

What Led to the Legislation?

Accutane, a powerful anti-acne drug, was shown to cause birth defects in the babies of mothers who used the drug. It also caused the spontaneous abortion of many babies. Other studies showed links to depression, psychosis, and suicide.

Key Points of the Legislation

This act was designed to create a mandatory program restricting the distribution of Accutane as well as its generic forms. It asked for a registry of all those involved in its distribution or use, public education about the drug, the prescribing of this drug only after other therapies have failed, the restriction of distribution to only medical offices and clinics, and quarterly reporting of all adverse effects.

THE COMBAT METHAMPHETAMINE EPIDEMIC ACT OF 2005

This act focused on the methamphetamine provisions of the Patriot Act extension, which itself was titled "The USA Patriot Act Improvements and Reauthorization Act." It was intended to stop the illegal use of the drug known as methamphetamine. Drug trafficking, used to financially support terrorism, is now regulated by this act, with stiff penalties to anyone found in violation. When methamphetamine is involved in terrorist activities in any way, the government can now confiscate the personal property of people involved. Other drugs, such as crack cocaine, are also named in this act.

Drug products that fall under this legislation must be kept behind a counter or in a locked case. The law limits sales of pure ephedrine or pseudoephedrine (which are precursors of methamphetamine) to only 9 grams per month per person. Customers purchasing these products must provide identification, and sign a sales log. Pharmacy technicians must assist the pharmacist in making sure that the sales log is maintained correctly, and that the products are placed out of reach of customers as required. Everyone involved in the selling of these products is required to be registered with the U.S. Attorney General's office, and trained about the provisions of the law.

What Led to the Legislation?

The use of methamphetamine and similar drugs has been on the increase, and their use has often crossed over the lines of other criminal activities, including terrorism. This act was intended to curb the manufacture and distribution of these drugs, as well as severely punish those individuals involved with them and other crimes.

Key Points of the Legislation

This act introduced safeguards to make ingredients used in the creation of methamphetamine and similar drugs harder to access. It also gave the government heightened powers to combat drug smuggling, manufacture, and distribution. The terrorism connection enables the government to pursue terrorists more effectively by using drug-related legislation to improve their law enforcement efforts.

REGULATORY AGENCIES

The following regulatory agencies each have specific activities that relate to public use and governmental control of specific substances. They are listed alphabetically by their abbreviations where applicable.

Bureau of Alcohol, Tobacco, and Firearms (ATF)

The ATF is dedicated to preventing terrorism, reducing violent crime, and protecting the U.S.A. It regulates alcohol, tobacco, firearms, and even explosives. The ATF also investigates acts of arson.

State Boards of Pharmacy (BOP)

The board of pharmacy in each state is designed to regulate and control the practice of pharmacy. These boards adopt laws that affect pharmacy practice. The focus of each board's activities is to protect the health of the public.

Centers for Medicare and Medicaid Service (CMS)

The CMS works to promote health-care coverage that is both effective and up-to-date. It also promotes quality health care for beneficiaries. The CMS intends to modernize the U.S. health-care system.

Drug Enforcement Agency (DEA)

The DEA strives to enforce controlled-substances legislation, and to bring offenders to justice, while also promoting the reduction of illicit substances. The DEA cooperates with local, regional, national, and international agencies in order to accomplish their mission. The DEA investigates and prosecutes major violators of controlled substance laws, with serious focus on those individuals or groups (including gangs) who use violence as part of their illegal activities. They also manage a national drug intelligence program that reaches into many other countries via liaisons with major crime-fighting agencies. The assets of violators are regularly seized by the DEA as part of their enforcement against illegal drug activities.

Department of Transportation (DOT)

The Department of Transportation regulates the safe transportation of hazardous and non-hazardous materials so that the general public and environment are protected from harm. The Hazardous Materials Transportation Uniform Safety Act of 1990 made regulations more constant and uniform between all 50 states.

Environmental Protection Agency (EPA)

The EPA strives to protect the environment and also the health of human beings. It develops and enforces environmental legislation, and offers grants to state environmental programs. It publishes information designed to educate the public and establish voluntary environmental partnerships and programs.

Food and Drug Administration (FDA)

The FDA was created from the Food, Drug, and Insecticide Administration in 1930. The FDA's intent is to promote public health. It controls the safety and effectiveness of foods, drugs, biological products, medical devices, cosmetics, and radioactive substances. It also provides information about better, safer, and more cost-effective products. The FDA should be notified when adverse reactions, problems with product quality, or product-use errors occur. The system that they have in place for this reporting is called "MedWatch." This system serves both health-care professionals and the public. Information about MedWatch and making reports to the FDA can be found at http://www.fda.gov (click on "Safety Alerts (MedWatch)" on the "Drugs" menu).

The Joint Commission on Accreditation of Health-care Organizations (JCAHO)

The Joint Commission accredits and certifies health-care organizations in the United States. While not actually a government agency, its ultimate goal is to improve the safety and quality of health care. The Joint Commission is an independent, not-for-profit organization that is recognized nationwide. It strives to continually improve the quality of its programs, so that accredited organizations may offer increased patient safety.

National Association of the Boards of Pharmacy (NABP)

The NABP assists its member boards and jurisdictions to protect public health by developing uniform standards. While not a government agency, the NABP also implements these standards to reduce potential harm to the public that may result because of the increasing complexities of medications and delivery systems.

Institutional Review Boards (IRB)

Institutional review boards are designed to oversee biomedical and behavioral research to protect the public. They can approve or reject new research, or even ask for modifications to the research. They are regulated by the Office for Human Research Protections (OHRP), which is part of the Department of Health and Human Services (HHS).

SUMMARY

Many laws and amendments were enacted over the past 100 years to shape the current Food, Drug, and Cosmetic Act. In the practice of pharmacy, the control of drugs is governed by laws, regulations, and standards. Pharmacy technicians should understand the different terminology used in the law, and which punishments may be given for certain violations.

The U.S. Congress passed the first important federal law governing pharmacy, the Pure Food and Drug Act, in 1906. Because of the tragedy involving sulfanilamide in 1937, which caused more than 100 patient deaths from the ingesting of Elixir Sulfanilamide, the Food, Drug, and Cosmetic Act was passed in 1938.

The Durham-Humphrey Amendment of 1951 prohibited dispensing of legend drugs without a prescription. The Federal Food, Drug, and Cosmetic Act was amended again with the Kefauver-Harris Amendment of 1962 to require that drug products, both prescription and non-prescription, must be effective as well as safe.

Since 1970, Congress has passed several important laws, including the Poison Prevention Packaging Act (to prevent and protect children from accidental poisoning through the use of child-resistant packaging), the Controlled Substances Act, and the Medical Device Amendment of 1976 (for the safety and effectiveness of life-sustaining and life-supporting devices). The Orphan Drug Act, passed in 1983, offers tax breaks and a 7-year monopoly on drug sales in order to induce companies to undertake the development and manufacturing of drugs used for rare diseases or conditions (such as the treatment of AIDS, cystic fibrosis, blepharospasm, and snake bites).

OBRA-90 was instituted to reduce Medicaid costs. Most significantly, it requires manufacturers to provide the lowest possible prices by rebating each state Medicaid agency the difference between the average price of a drug and the lowest available price. It also requires drug use evaluation (DUE) and the offer to counsel patients in order to make sure that drug therapy is as safe and as effective as it can be. The FDA's Safe Medical Devices Act (SMDA) requires all medical devices to be tracked and records maintained for durable medical equipment. The Anabolic Steroids Control Act allowed the CSA to regulate anabolic steroids, which are often used illegally by athletes to promote muscle growth.

The Americans with Disabilities Act (ADA) was established to prohibit discrimination against disabled persons. The Dietary Supplement Health and Education Act controls many different supplements, including amino acids, herbs and botanicals, some hormones, minerals, and vitamins. The Health Insurance Portability and Accountability Act (HIPAA) was designed to regulate patient privacy, security, and transaction standards relating to electronic health records. Separate acts were established that modernized the FDA, as well as adding Medicare Part D. The Combat Methamphetamine Epidemic Act was intended to stop the use of illegal drugs such as methamphetamine, crack cocaine, and other drugs, especially related to how their sale is often used to finance terrorism.

SETTING THE SCENE

The following discussion and responses relate to the opening "Setting the Scene" scenario:

- The pharmacy technician must not package the prescription in a non-child-resistant container.

- Both the pharmacy technician and the pharmacist ignored the Poison Prevention Packaging Act of 1970. This act requires that child-resistant containers must be provided unless an adult patient specifically requests non-child-resistant containers.

- Both are responsible for this error, but mainly the pharmacist, who supervises the technician.

REVIEW QUESTIONS

Multiple Choice

1. The Food, Drug, and Cosmetic Act was passed in:

    A. 1906
    B. 1914
    C. 1938
    D. 1962

2. The Harrison Narcotics Tax Act was part of:

    A. the Internal Revenue Code
    B. toxicity tests after the sulfanilamide tragedy
    C. internal regulations to create classifications of prescriptions
    D. toxicity tests after the thalidomide tragedy

3. The labeling of a medication in a way that is false or misleading is referred to as:

    A. adulteration
    B. distribution
    C. fraud
    D. misbranding

4. The first U.S. act prohibiting the interstate distribution or sale of adulterated or misbranded food and drugs was passed in:

    A. 1906
    B. 1912
    C. 1914
    D. 1938

5. The FDA is a branch of which department, that controls all drugs for legal use?

    A. U.S. Department of Health
    B. U.S. Department of Health and Human Services
    C. U.S. Department of Agriculture
    D. U.S. Department of Labor

6. Which of the following acts was designed to protect the public health by requiring that only safe and properly labeled drugs may be introduced into interstate commerce?

    A. the Durham-Humphrey Amendment
    B. the Kefauver-Harris Amendment
    C. the Harrison Narcotics Tax Act
    D. the Pure Food and Drug Act

7. In 1937, the Massengill Company introduced Elixir Sulfanilamide into the market, which contained a solution containing which of the following substances?

    A. glycerin
    B. chloroform
    C. diethylene glycol
    D. methyl alcohol

8. Which act required that pharmaceutical manufacturers file a New Drug Application with the FDA?

    A. Durham-Humphrey Amendment
    B. Kefauver-Harris Amendment
    C. Poison Prevention Packaging Act
    D. Food, Drug, and Cosmetic Act

9. Which of the following acts offers federal financial incentives to commercial and nonprofit organizations for the development of drugs?

    A. Medical Device Amendment
    B. Drug Listing Act
    C. Orphan Drug Act
    D. Poison Prevention Packaging Act

10. Which of the following laws was passed to establish clear criteria for classifications of legend and OTC drugs?

    A. Kefauver-Harris Amendment
    B. Durham-Humphrey Amendment
    C. Harrison Narcotics Tax Act
    D. Pure Food and Drug Act

11. When patients agree to be part of a study that tests a new drug, they must be thoroughly educated about its possible medical risks. This is referred to as:

    A. informed consent
    B. a black box warning
    C. post drug approval
    D. drug review

12. Orphan drugs are used for all of the following disorders or conditions, except:

    A. cystic fibrosis
    B. hepatitis A
    C. blepharospasm
    D. snake bite

13. Before the FDA prevented thalidomide from reaching the U.S. market, it had been tested around the world as:

    A. a tranquilizer
    B. a sedative
    C. an anti-nauseant during pregnancy
    D. all of the above

14. The five controlled substance "schedules" were established by the:

    A. Harrison Narcotics Tax Act
    B. Comprehensive Drug Abuse Prevention and Control Act
    C. Drug Regulation Reform Act
    D. Drug Listing Act

15.   Which of the following acts requires that most legend drugs be packaged in child-resistant containers?

A.   Drug Listing Act
B.   Food, Drug, and Cosmetic Act
C.   Harrison Narcotics Tax Act
D.   Poison Prevention Packaging Act

Fill in the Blank

1.   The act that restricted the sale of drugs by requiring a prescription was the _____.

2.   The Kefauver-Harris Amendment required that drug products must be _____ and _____, as well as _____.

3.   The act that required employers to provide safe and healthy working environments was known as _____.

4.   The FDA uses a special code to maintain a database of drugs; this code is made up of numbers that represent usage, manufacturer, drug product, and type of packaging. This code is known as the _____.

5.   The act that regulates solid waste landfills to protect humans, animals, and the environment is known as the _____.

6.   The Drug Regulation Reform Act and its provisions were designed to encourage _____ FDA regulation of the _____ industry.

7.   The drug that was recalled due to thousands of lawsuits related to fatal arrhythmias and heart diseases was called _____.

8.   Orphan drugs are used to treat diseases affecting fewer than _____ people in the U.S.

9.   OBRA-90 requires that manufacturers provide reduced Medicaid costs by rebating the difference between a drug's _____ price and the _____ available price.

10.   The organization that accredits health-care organizations is known as _____.

CASE STUDY

A pharmacy technician asks the pharmacist if it is suitable to substitute Fiorinal No. 3 for Sedapap, which was prescribed, because of the nearly identical chemical properties of the two drugs. He explains to the pharmacist that the pharmacy is out of Sedapap, and that the prescribing physician did indicate that a suitable substitution medication was allowed. After taking the Fiorinal No. 3, which contains codeine (to which the patient is allergic), she is hospitalized after going into anaphylactic shock. It is later found that Fiorinal No. 3 (a Schedule III drug because of its codeine content) is vastly different than the drug simply referred to as Fiorinal, a non-narcotic agonist analgesic.

1. Is this error the fault of the pharmacy technician only?

2. Is it the fault of the physician?

3. What are the potential outcomes of this error?

RELATED INTERNET SITES

At the Web sites listed, search for the various laws outlined in the chapter.

http://aspe.hhs.gov

http://content.healthaffairs.org/cgi/reprint/10/1/192.pdf

http://depts.washington.edu/hiprc; **click on "Best Practices" and then "Poisoning"**

http://library.findlaw.com

http://www.accutanerecalls.com

http://www.ada.gov

http://www.annals.org

http://www.atf.treas.gov

http://www.cancer.gov

http://www.cfsan.fda.gov; **click on "laws enforced by the FDA"**

http://www.cms.hhs.gov

http://www.dea.gov

http://www.dol.gov

http://www.drugrecalls.com

http://www.epa.gov

http://www.fda.gov

http://www.fda.gov/medwatch

http://www.hhs.gov

http://www.jointcommission.org

http://www.osha.gov

http://www.usdoj.gov/dea/pubs/abuse/chart.htm

http://www.uspharmd.com

http://www.whitehouse.gov

REFERENCES

Abood, R. (2005). *Pharmacy Practice and the Law* (4th ed.). Jones and Bartlett.

Reiss, B. S., & Hall, G. D. (2006). *Guide to Federal Pharmacy Law* (5th ed.). Apothecary Press.

Strandberg, K. M. (2002). *Essentials of Law and Ethics for Pharmacy Technicians.* CRC Press.

Comprehensive Drug Abuse and Prevention Control Act: A Closer Look

OBJECTIVES

Upon completion of this chapter, the reader should be able to:

1. Describe Schedule I versus Schedule II drugs.
2. Identify the significance of each controlled substance Schedule.
3. Distinguish between prescription drugs, nonprescription drugs, and controlled substances.
4. Explain the Controlled Substances Act and Schedule drugs.
5. Describe labeling of controlled substances.
6. Explain the importance of recording refills for controlled substances.
7. Describe the importance of record keeping for controlled substances.
8. Explain DEA Forms 41, 106, and 222.
9. Describe the process of returning controlled substances.
10. Identify state and federal law regarding controlled substances.

KEY TERMS

Anabolic steroids – Schedule III controlled substances (either drugs or hormonal substances) that are often misused by athletes seeking to enhance their bulk (by increasing muscle mass) and physical prowess.

"C" symbol – A marking that indicates a controlled substance, and is printed on a drug's label, its box, and/or its packaging insert.

Data processing system – An alternative, computerized method for the storage and retrieval of prescription refill information for controlled substances in Schedules III and IV.

Drug Enforcement Administration (DEA) – The bureau within the United States Department of Justice primarily responsible for policing federal laws that concern controlled substances. In addition to investigating the sellers, producers, and smugglers of illicit drugs, the DEA also monitors physician prescribing patterns and pharmacy purchases.

Facsimile – A copy of an official document (such as a prescription or medication order) that is commonly transmitted via fax machine.

Schedules – The five classifications of controlled substances, with the drugs having the highest potential for abuse and no medical use listed in Schedule I, and those with progressively less abuse potential listed in Schedules II, III, IV, and V.

SETTING THE SCENE

Anthony, a pharmacy technician who has been working for 10 years in a retail pharmacy, has authority over inventory management. One day, he fills out a Form 222 to order two different Schedule II drugs, without informing his pharmacist. He does not have Power of Attorney authorizing him to be able to sign for Schedule II drugs. He signs the form himself and faxes it to his supplier. The supplier calls the pharmacist and asks for an explanation as to why an unauthorized signature appears on the form. The pharmacist questions Anthony about these events.

Critical Thinking

- What did Anthony do wrong?

- Is his job in jeopardy because of this situation?

- Briefly explain the DEA's procedures related to ordering Schedule II drugs.

OVERVIEW

The **Drug Enforcement Administration (DEA)** was established in 1973 as part of the Department of Justice to enforce federal laws regarding the use of illegal drugs. According to the federal Controlled Substances Act (CSA), drugs or other substances that have the potential for illegal use (and abuse) must be included in the controlled substances list. Any new drugs with similar action to drugs already on the controlled substances list are also considered to have the same potential for abuse.

Pharmacy technicians must be familiar with the Comprehensive Drug Abuse and Prevention Control Act. They should understand its guidelines concerning controlled substances, their storage, security, and keeping of controlled substance records. Federal and state laws require all personnel, including pharmacy technicians, to help in the management of controlled substances located in the workplace. They must take precautions to monitor patient drug use, maintain correct records (as required by law), and report any known or suspected theft or diversion of drugs.

CLASSIFICATION OF SCHEDULED DRUGS

The drugs that come under the jurisdiction of the Controlled Substances Act (CSA) have been categorized according to their potential for abuse and their addictive abilities. They are divided into five schedules, which range from Schedule I (illegal drugs and those that cannot be prescribed) to Schedule V (drugs that have the least potential for addiction and abuse). Scheduling requests may be initiated by the Department of Health and Human Services (DHHS), by the DEA, or by petition of a manufacturer, medical society, pharmaceutical association, public interest group, or an individual citizen.

The states with the harshest penalties for controlled substance convictions are New York and Michigan. Because of drug laws initiated by Nelson Rockefeller, drug convictions involving Schedule I or II controlled substances brought punishments nearly as severe as those allotted for murder. This included life imprisonment in certain circumstances. It is important to note that when a state law conflicts with the federal government's position concerning a specific drug, the stricter law takes precedence. Discrepancies should be handled by contacting the closest DEA office to determine your state's regulations, as well as the federal government's regulations concerning any controlled substance in question.

Schedule I

Schedule I agents are not accepted for medical use in the United States. They possess an extremely high potential for abuse. Properly registered people may use Schedule I substances for research purposes. Examples of Schedule I drugs include: opiates, opium derivatives (such as heroin), crystal methamphetamine, hallucinogens (such as lysergic acid diethylamide [LSD], marijuana, and mescaline), peyote, stimulants such as methcathinone, hashish, crack cocaine, depressants such as methaqualone and gamma-hydroxy butyrate (GHB), and dihydromorphine.

Schedule II

Schedule II agents have medical uses, but also a high abuse potential, with severe physical or psychological dependence. The broad categories of Schedule II drugs include opiates and opium derivatives, derivatives of cocoa leaves, and certain central nervous system stimulants and depressants. Examples of Schedule II drugs include: opiates and opioids [narcotics] (such as opium, fentanyl, hydromorphone, methadone, morphine, meperidine, oxycodone, and oxymorphone), stimulants (such as amphetamine and methylphenidate), and depressants (such as amobarbital, pentobarbital, secobarbital, and various combinations of depressants).

The quantity of the substance in a drug product often determines the schedule that will control it. For example, amphetamines and codeine usually are classified in Schedule II. However, Schedules III and IV control specific products containing smaller quantities of Schedule II substances, most often in combination with a non-controlled substance.

Schedule III

These agents have accepted medical uses, with less abuse potential than Schedule I and II drugs. Anabolic steroids were and are misused by athletes seeking to enhance their bulk and physical prowess. Competitive and peer pressure to use these drugs is constant. In 1988, Congress responded by amending the Food, Drug, and Cosmetic Act, declaring that distribution or possession with intent to distribute for human use, *other than for the treatment of disease upon the order of a physician,* was punishable by not more than three years' imprisonment and/or a fine, or both. If the person possessed such drugs as anabolic steroids with the intent to distribute them to a minor under 18 years of age, the penalty was increased to 6 years of imprisonment.

In 1990, anabolic steroids were added to Schedule III as controlled substances. Some feel that anabolic steroids were swept into the controlled substance category simply to take advantage of the broad enforcement arm of the DEA as well as the penalties that attach to the violation of the CSA. Other examples of Schedule III drugs include: nalorphine, buprenorphone, buprenorphone with naloxone, acetaminophen with codeine, aspirin with codeine, acetaminophen with hydrocodone, ibuprofen with hydrocodone, butabarbital, and other barbiturates combined with non-control drugs such as aspirin.

Focus On...

Anabolic Steroids

Anabolic steroids are substances that are chemically and pharmacologically related to testosterone (other than estrogens, progestin, and corticosteroids), and promote muscle growth.

Schedule IV

The abuse potential for Schedule IV drugs is less than those in Schedule III. However, abuse of Schedule IV drugs can still lead to physical or psychological dependency. Schedule IV drugs are generally the long-acting barbiturates, certain hypnotics, and minor tranquilizers. For all practical purposes, there are no regulatory differences between Schedules III and IV. Examples of Schedule IV drugs include: benzodiazepines, fenfluramine, propoxyphene (alone or in combination with acetaminophen), phenobarbital, chlordiazepoxide, alprazolam, ethinamate, diethylpropion, temazepam, meprobamate, clonazepam, and diazepam.

Schedule V

Schedule V agents have the lowest abuse potential of the controlled substances and consist of preparations containing limited quantities of certain narcotic drugs, generally used for antitussive and antidiarrheal purposes. Examples of Schedule V drugs include: antidiarrheals, analgesics, cough syrups that contain codeine, diphenoxylate mixtures, certain strengths of opium mixtures, pseudoephedrine, and phenergan with codeine. While a few Schedule V drugs do not require a prescription, there are still requirements for their sale. As controlled substances, they may be sold OTC but the sale must be recorded in a log book, including information about the person making the purchase, the quantity, and strength of the drug. The pharmacy's name and date, and the pharmacist's initials must be placed on the bottle containing the medication. Of the Schedule V drugs, phenobarbital, various prescription cough syrups containing codeine, and acetaminophen with codeine elixir all require prescriptions. Table 4-1 shows drug schedules and some examples.

TABLE 4-1 Drug Schedules

Schedule	Abuse Potential	Examples
I (No prescription permitted)	High No accepted medical use	Fenethylline (also spelled "phenethylline") • Hallucinogens • Hashish • Heroin • Lysergic acid diethylamide (LSD) • Marijuana • Methaqualone (Quaalude®) • Peyote
II (No refills permitted without a new written prescription)	High Accepted medical use	Amphetamines • Barbiturates (short-acting) • Cocaine • Hydromorphone HCl (Dilaudid®) • Morphine • Narcotics • Opium
III (5 refills permitted within 6 months)	Moderate Accepted medical use	Anabolic Steroids • Barbiturates (moderate-acting) • Butabarbital (Butisol®) • Codeine mixtures (most of them) • Glutethimide
IV (5 refills permitted within 6 months)	Low Accepted medical use	Alprazolam (Xanax®) • Chloral hydrate (Noctec®) • Diazepam (Valium®) • Pentazocine HCl (Talwin®)

(continued)

TABLE 4-1   Drug Schedules (*continued*)

Schedule	Abuse Potential	Examples
V (No prescription required for individuals who are 18 or older for most of these drugs; however, they may only be sold at pharmacies and require pharmacist involvement in their sale)	Low Accepted medical use	Cough syrups with codeine (Cheracol® with codeine) • Guaifenesin mixtures (such as Naldecon Dx®) • Lomotil® Parepectolin® • Robitussin AC® • • Pseudoephedrine

DEA REGISTRATION FOR CONTROLLED SUBSTANCES

Individuals who manufacture, dispense, or distribute any controlled substance are obligated to register with the DEA, unless they are exempted. Pharmacy registrations are issued for 3 years. A DEA number must be assigned to those who are registered under the law as manufacturers, distributors, wholesalers, and practitioners, such as physicians, dentists, veterinarians, scientists, pharmacies, and hospitals. Each state regulates which medical professionals may prescribe controlled substances. If an individual is authorized by his or her state to order controlled substances, he or she may apply for a DEA number. Some states allow Certified Nurse Practitioners to prescribe, and a few states allow optometrists to prescribe.

All pharmacies must have a valid DEA registration, which grants them the authority to handle controlled substances as specified in their registration documents. This is determined by both state and federal laws. To register, new pharmacy applicants are required to complete DEA Form 224 and submit it to the following address: DEA, Registration Unit, Central Station, PO Box 28083, Washington, D.C. 20038-8083. DEA registrations must be renewed every three years.

If the DEA registrant is not the same person who controls the pharmacy's day-to-day operations, or who orders controlled substances, a Power of Attorney may be used, which requires two signatures in order to be valid. Records of transactions made using a Power of Attorney must be kept on file for 2 years.

A DEA number can be checked for legitimacy in two ways. The first method is a simple calculation that checks its authenticity. A DEA number is made up of a two-letter prefix, followed by seven digits. The first letter is an "A" if the practitioner began practice before 1988, and a "B" if they began practice later. The second letter comes from the practitioner's last name – if the last name is "Smith," it would be an "S." To verify accuracy of the digits, add up the first, third, and fifth numbers. Then add up the second, fourth, and sixth numbers, after which you multiply this result by two. Add this new total to the total of the first, third, and fifth numbers. Look at this new total – the last digit of this total will be the same as the seventh digit in the DEA number.

Focus On...

Verifying a DEA number

Dr. Smith's DEA number is: BS3076216. Using the instructions indicated above, to check the digits you would do the following:

> *Add the first, third, and fifth digits (3 + 7 + 2 = 12).*
>
> *Add the second, fourth, and sixth digits (0 + 6 + 1 = 7).*
>
> *Multiply by 2 (7 × 2 = 14).*
>
> *Add the first total to the second total (12 + 14 = 26).*
>
> *The last digit of this total, which is a **6**, is the same as the seventh digit in the*
>
> *DEA number "BS307621**6**".*

The second method is online verification for the actual DEA registrant – this provides the registrant's name, DEA number, and DEA address of record. Data on registrants is updated monthly by the Department of Justice. Health care providers and other entities can subscribe to various systems to verify DEA numbers. An example of one of these online services is located at: www.dealookup.com/home.asp.

Focus On...

DEA Registration

When a DEA registration is terminated, revoked, or suspended for any reason, all unused DEA forms must be returned to the closest DEA office.

> *DEA Form 224 must be used for pharmacy registration. It must be renewed every three years. See Figure 4-1.*

(continued)

Form-224

APPLICATION FOR REGISTRATION
Under the Controlled Substances Act

APPROVED OMB NO 1117-0014
FORM DEA-224 (10-06)
Previous editions are obsolete

INSTRUCTIONS

Save time - apply on-line at www.deadiversion.usdoj.gov

1. To apply by mail complete this application. Keep a copy for your records.
2. Print clearly, using black or blue ink, or use a typewriter.
3. Mail this form to the address provided in Section 7 or use enclosed envelope.
4. Include the correct payment amount. FEE IS NON-REFUNDABLE.
5. If you have any questions call 800-882-9539 prior to submitting your application.

IMPORTANT: DO NOT SEND THIS APPLICATION **AND** APPLY ON-LINE.

DEA OFFICIAL USE :

Do you have other DEA registration numbers?

☐ NO   ☐ YES

MAIL-TO ADDRESS   Please print mailing address changes to the right of the address in this box.

FEE FOR THREE (3) YEARS IS $551
FEE IS NON-REFUNDABLE

SECTION 1   APPLICANT IDENTIFICATION

☐ Individual Registration   ☐ Business Registration

Name 1   (Last Name of individual -OR- Business or Facility Name)

Name 2   (First Name and Middle Name of individual - OR- Continuation of business name)

Street Address Line 1 (if applying for fee exemption, this must be address of the fee exempt institution)

Address Line 2

City   State   Zip Code

Business Phone Number   Point of Contact

Business Fax Number   Email Address

DEBT COLLECTION INFORMATION

Mandatory pursuant to Debt Collection Improvements Act

Social Security Number (*if registration is for individual*)

Provide SSN or TIN.
See additional information
note #3 on page 4.

Tax Identification Number (*if registration is for business*)

FOR Practitioner or MLP ONLY:

Professional Degree :
select from list only

Professional School :

Year of Graduation :

National Provider Identification:

Date of Birth (*MM-DD-YYYY*):

M M   D D   Y Y Y Y

SECTION 2
BUSINESS ACTIVITY

Check one business activity box only

☐ Central Fill Pharmacy
☐ Retail Pharmacy
☐ Nursing Home
☐ Automated Dispensing System

☐ Practitioner (DDS, DMD, DO, DPM, DVM, MD or PHD)
☐ Practitioner Military (DDS, DMD, DO, DPM, DVM, MD or PHD)
☐ Mid-level Practitioner (MLP) (DOM, HMD, MP, ND, NP, OD, PA, or RPH)
☐ Euthanasia Technician

☐ Ambulance Service
☐ Animal Shelter
☐ Hospital/Clinic
☐ Teaching Institution

FOR Automated Dispensing System (ADS) ONLY:

DEA Registration # of Retail Pharmacy for this ADS

An ADS is automatically fee-exempt. Skip Section 6 and Section 7 on page 2. You must attach a notorized affidavit.

SECTION 3
DRUG SCHEDULES

Check all that apply

☐ Schedule II Narcotic
☐ Schedule II Non-Narcotic

☐ Schedule III Narcotic
☐ Schedule III Non-Narcotic

☐ Schedule IV
☐ Schedule V

☐ Check this box if you require official order forms - for purchase or transfer of schedule 2 narcotic and/or schedule 2 non-narcotic controlled substances.

NEW - Page 1

Figure 4-1 DEA Form 224.

SECTION 4

STATE LICENSE(S)

You MUST be currently authorized to prescribe, distribute, dispense, conduct research, or otherwise handle the controlled substances in the schedules for which you are applying under the laws of the **state** or jurisdiction in which you are operating or propose to operate.

Be sure to include both state license numbers if applicable

State License Number (required)

Expiration Date (required)   /   /
MM - DD - YYYY

What state was this license issued in? _____

State Controlled Substance License Number (if required)

Expiration Date   /   /
MM - DD - YYYY

What state was this license issued in? _____

SECTION 5

LIABILITY

IMPORTANT

All questions in this section must be answered.

1. Has the applicant ever been **convicted of a crime** in connection with controlled substance(s) under state or federal law, or is any such action pending?   **YES NO** ☐ ☐

   Date(s) of incident MM-DD-YYYY: ☐☐—☐☐—☐☐☐☐

2. Has the applicant ever surrendered (for cause) or had a **federal** controlled substance registration revoked, suspended, restricted, or denied, or is any such action pending?   **YES NO** ☐ ☐

   Date(s) of incident MM-DD-YYYY: ☐☐—☐☐—☐☐☐☐

3. Has the applicant ever surrendered (for cause) or had a **state** professional license or controlled substance registration revoked, suspended, denied, restricted, or placed on probation, or is any such action pending?   **YES NO** ☐ ☐

   Date(s) of incident MM-DD-YYYY: ☐☐—☐☐—☐☐☐☐

4. If the applicant is a **corporation** (other than a corporation whose stock is owned and traded by the public), association, partnership, or pharmacy, has any officer, partner, stockholder, or proprietor been **convicted of a crime** in connection with controlled substance(s) under state or federal law, or ever surrendered, for cause, or had a **federal** controlled substance registration revoked, suspended, restricted, denied, or ever had a **state** professional license or controlled substance registration revoked, suspended, denied, restricted or placed on probation, or is any such action pending?   **YES NO** ☐ ☐

   Date(s) of incident MM-DD-YYYY: ☐☐—☐☐—☐☐☐☐   *Note: If question 4 does not apply to you, be sure to mark 'NO'. It will slow down processing of your application if you leave it blank.*

EXPLANATION OF "YES" ANSWERS

Applicants who have answered "YES" to any of the four questions above **must provide a statement to explain each "YES" answer.**

Use this space or attach a separate sheet and return with application

Liability question # _____   Location(s) of incident: _____

Nature of incident:

Disposition of incident:

SECTION 6   EXEMPTION FROM APPLICATION FEE

☐ Check this box if the applicant is a federal, state, or local government official or institution. Does not apply to contractor-operated institutions.

Business or Facility Name of Fee Exempt Institution. **Be sure to enter the address of this exempt institution in Section 1.**

The undersigned hereby certifies that the applicant named hereon is a federal, state or local government official or institution, and is exempt from payment of the application fee.

FEE EXEMPT CERTIFIER

Provide the name and phone number of the certifying official

Signature of certifying official (**other than applicant**)   Date

Print or type name and title of certifying official   Telephone No. (required for verification)

SECTION 7

METHOD OF PAYMENT

Check one form of payment only

☐ Check   Make check payable to: **Drug Enforcement Administration**
See page 4 of instructions for important information.

☐ American Express   ☐ Discover   ☐ Master Card   ☐ Visa

Credit Card Number   Expiration Date

Sign if paying by credit card

Signature of Card Holder

Printed Name of Card Holder

Mail this form with payment to:

U.S. Department of Justice
Drug Enforcement Administration
P.O. Box 28083
Washington, DC 20038-8083

FEE IS NON-REFUNDABLE

SECTION 8

APPLICANT'S SIGNATURE

Sign in ink

I certify that the foregoing information furnished on this application is true and correct.

Signature of applicant (sign in ink)   Date

Print or type name and title of applicant

WARNING: Section 843(a)(4)(A) of Title 21, United States Code states that any person who knowingly or intentionally furnishes false or fraudulent information in the application is subject to imprisonment for not more than four years, a fine of not more than $30,000, or both.

NEW - Page 2

Figure 4-1 DEA Form 224 *(continued).*

Registration Certificate

Falsification of an application will result in the suspension or revocation of the applicant's registration by the DEA. If the applicant has a previous felony conviction related to controlled substances, a suspended registration, or a suspended state license, the applicant will no longer be allowed to dispense controlled substances.

Except in emergency situations, registrants are assured of a hearing and due process of law prior to suspension or revocation of registration. In addition, anyone who discontinues his or her business or professional practice, ends his or her legal existence, or dies, automatically has his or her registration terminated.

Security of Personnel

Background checks should be carried out for all potential employees who will work in the proximity of controlled substances. Interviewees must supply truthful information about past convictions or criminal charges against them. They must also answer questions about any illegal drug use. Lying or providing incomplete answers concerning these topics may lead to future legal situations between the prospective employee and employer, and even between the prospective employee and the state.

You Be the Judge

Glenn, a pharmacy technician who has been working for a year, was required because of new pharmacy rules to take drug-screening tests upon starting his second year at work. The new rules also required a full background check to be made. When Glenn's test results were returned, he had a positive result for cocaine in his system, and the background check revealed that he had a previous conviction for drug possession. In your judgment, what will be the result of Glenn's positive drug test and his background check?

REGULATION OF CONTROLLED SUBSTANCES

There are specific CSA regulations that govern the record keeping, physician and pharmacy registrations, and inventory concerning controlled substances. All scheduled drugs used in any ambulatory care setting must have complete and accurate records kept concerning their purchase, storage, management, and distribution.

Focus On...

State Law and Controlled Substances

State governments regulate certain substances not controlled at the federal level. These include substances such as: toluene, amyl or butyl nitrite, and nitrous oxide. Many states enforce age limits concerning the sale of products that contain these substances.

Controlled substances may also be regulated by individual states, and pharmacists must comply with the regulations of their state regarding the handling of controlled substances. Because of this, pharmacy technicians must understand their state's legal requirements. Specific guidelines for controlled substance prescriptions include:

- Prescription forms must be written in ink or typed, except for hospice and nursing home prescriptions, which may be faxed to the pharmacy – the fax may be used as the hard copy
- Federal law does not require a physical prescription, but individual states may choose to do so
- They must include the date prescribed, patient's name and address, and physician's DEA number
- Amount prescribed should be written out in order to avoid errors – "fifteen" should be used instead of "15"
- The physician must physically sign every written controlled substance prescription, but can verbally order Schedule III, IV, and V controlled substances

Focus On...

Roles of Pharmacy Technicians

According to individual state law, pharmacy technicians may count scheduled drugs, do inventory, and record keeping. In many states, they can only have access to the pharmacy safe, room, or cabinet that contains scheduled drugs if supervised by the pharmacist, and the pharmacist must keep the keys to the safe. Federal regulations do not actually restrict access to controlled substance containment areas by pharmacy technicians. Only a licensed pharmacist is able to dispense scheduled drugs.

ORDERING CONTROLLED SUBSTANCES

DEA Form 222 is used to order controlled substances from Schedules I or II. This form, which is filled out in triplicate, may be ordered from the DEA by phone, mail, or online, and is free of charge. However, the DEA is changing Form 222, including enhanced security features. It is now being provided as a single-sheet document, which is easier to use and reduces paperwork. Instead of using carbon paper between three separate sheets of paper, it now may simply be photocopied, with the copies being distributed in the same manner in which the previous triplicate version was distributed. Anyone attempting to order controlled substances must have a DEA license. DEA Form 222 is not used when ordering Schedule III, IV, or V substances, which can be ordered directly from manufacturers and other registrants.

Focus On...

Ordering Controlled Substances

After a pharmacy orders and receives Schedule III, IV, or V drugs, the invoice must be confirmed as accurate and dated. Though not required, it is often stamped with a red "C" to signify "controlled substance." The invoice or packing slip must be kept in a separate, secure location in the pharmacy for a minimum of 2 years.

Form 222 requires the person ordering the substances to supply the following information: company name and address, ordering date, number of packages of each item, size of package of each item, name of each item, signature of purchaser or his or her attorney or agent, and DEA registration number. It is important to note that not every pharmacist in a given pharmacy can sign DEA 222 forms. There must be someone dedicated to do this or a Power of Attorney in place. A maximum of 10 different items may be ordered on one form, with 1 item per numbered line. After all the items are entered, the DEA registrant must notate the number of lines completed using a designated space on the left side of the form – this helps to assure that no other person enters any substances onto the form after it is completed. This form should never be signed or dated prior to ordering in order to avoid fraudulent activities. Each book of ordering forms contains seven sets of these forms. A pharmacy may have no more than six books of forms at a given time, unless they can prove the need to have more.

Focus On...

Storage of Form 222

Copies of DEA Form 222 must be kept separate from the business records of the pharmacy. Unused copies of this form must be shown to the DEA inspectors if they arrive to conduct a DEA inspection.

When the supplier receives each form and processes the order, they must add the following information to the form: his or her DEA registration number, the national drug code of each item, an indication of the packaging being shipped, and the date of each shipment. In most states, the supplier keeps a copy of the purchasing company or individual's DEA certificate on file prior to shipping any order. This is good practice, but not required by federal regulations. The supplier can only ship to the purchaser's address that is listed on both the Form 222 and his or her DEA certificate. Form 222 is shown in Figure 4-2.

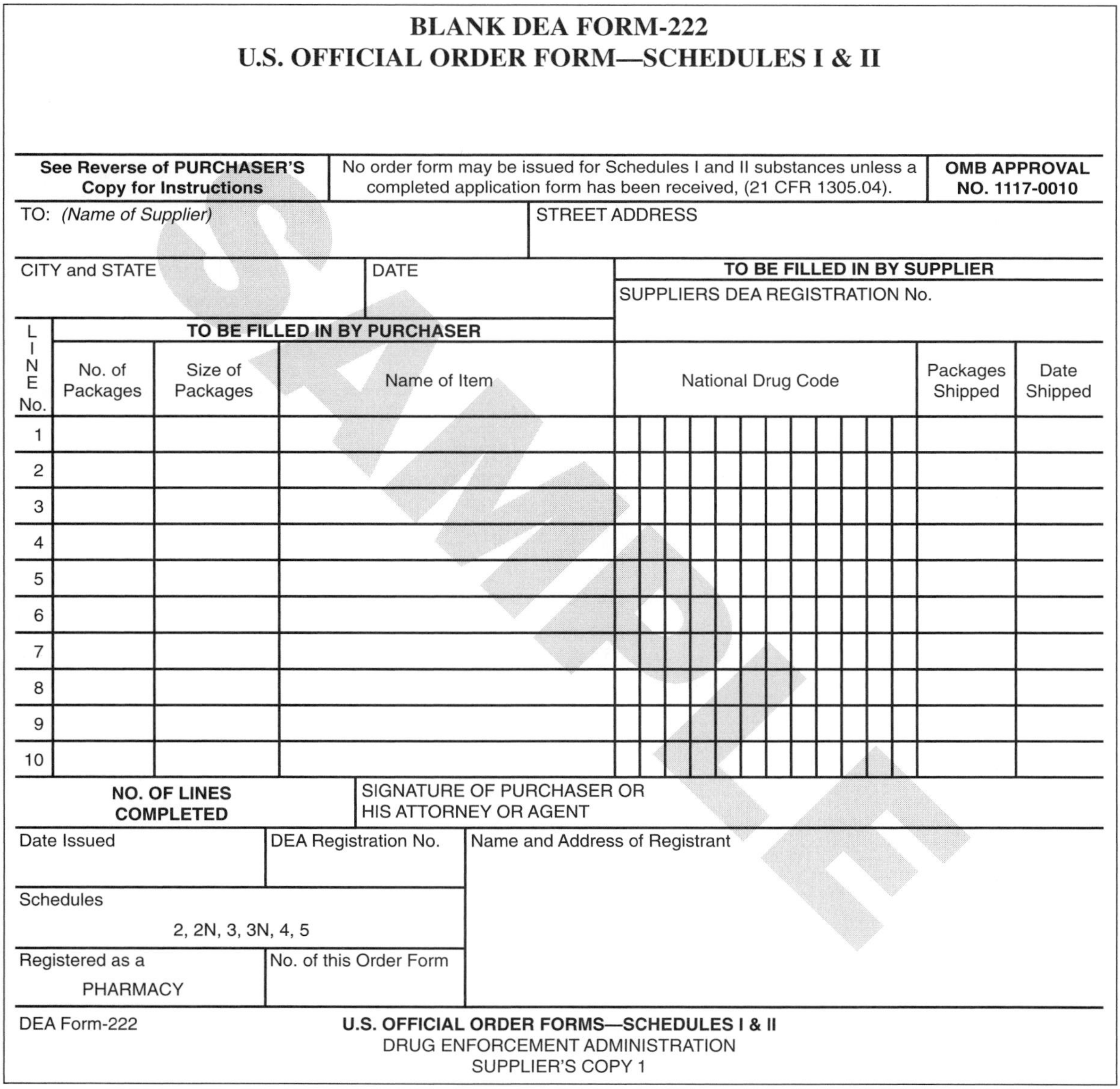

BLANK DEA FORM-222
U.S. OFFICIAL ORDER FORM—SCHEDULES I & II

See Reverse of PURCHASER'S Copy for Instructions	No order form may be issued for Schedules I and II substances unless a completed application form has been received, (21 CFR 1305.04).	OMB APPROVAL NO. 1117-0010

TO: *(Name of Supplier)*	STREET ADDRESS

CITY and STATE	DATE	TO BE FILLED IN BY SUPPLIER SUPPLIERS DEA REGISTRATION No.

LINE No.	TO BE FILLED IN BY PURCHASER					
	No. of Packages	Size of Packages	Name of Item	National Drug Code	Packages Shipped	Date Shipped
1						
2						
3						
4						
5						
6						
7						
8						
9						
10						

NO. OF LINES COMPLETED	SIGNATURE OF PURCHASER OR HIS ATTORNEY OR AGENT

Date Issued	DEA Registration No.	Name and Address of Registrant
Schedules 2, 2N, 3, 3N, 4, 5		
Registered as a PHARMACY	No. of this Order Form	

DEA Form-222

U.S. OFFICIAL ORDER FORMS—SCHEDULES I & II
DRUG ENFORCEMENT ADMINISTRATION
SUPPLIER'S COPY 1

Figure 4-2 DEA Form 222.

Focus On...

Form 222

When Form 222 is used, the first copy stays with the pharmaceutical supplier. The second copy goes to the DEA from the pharmaceutical supplier. The third copy remains with the pharmacy or entity that is ordering the pharmaceutical.

If a Form 222 is defective, or contains errors or omissions, corrections may be made only under these circumstances: the drug's name is misspelled, the date of the order is missing, the package size is missing, the strength of the drug is missing, the number of line items completed is missing, or if the items are placed in incorrect locations on the order form. Other than the above items, the order cannot be processed without a correct, new order form being submitted. Suppliers are instructed not to fill any order if the Form 222 is illegible, not endorsed (signed), or shows signs of being changed, erased, or altered.

Partial filling of a Form 222 order is allowed, but the balance of the order must be supplied within 60 days of the original order date.

Focus On...

Right to Refuse to Fill an Order

A supplier can refuse to fill an order for any reason and does not have to explain why fulfillment of the order is being refused. They only have to state that the order is not acceptable. A new order form can be submitted with all of the correct information included, but the returned order form must be filed and cannot be reused.

What Would You Do?

Joe, a pharmacist, gave a list of 13 Schedule II drugs to Betty so that she could write them onto a DEA Form 222. Betty wrote all 13 items on the 10-line form so that Joe could then sign it. Joe told her she would have to redo the form. What should Betty have done in this situation?

Electronic ordering is also available by using an electronic version of Form 222 called "e222." The use of e222 helps to prevent illegal ordering of controlled substances, because identifiers are used that make it very difficult for any non-authorized person to use this mode of ordering. The Web site used for electronic ordering is: http://www.deadiversion.usdoj.gov. While the use of e222 is not required, it is suggested over using the traditional paper forms because of the potential reduction in fraudulent activities.

When using e222, the following information is required: a unique number that the purchaser has created for themselves, the supplier's name/address/DEA number, the date the order is signed, the name of the controlled substance(s), the NDC number, the quantity (in a single package or container), and the number of packages or containers ordered. The "digital certificate" that is attached to the order provides the following: the purchaser's name/registered location/DEA number, his or her business activities, and his or her authorized schedules.

PRESCRIPTIONS FOR CONTROLLED SUBSTANCES

A practitioner must issue a prescription for a controlled substance for a valid medical purpose. If a practitioner attempts to re-supply an office stock by writing prescriptions for such a purpose, it is a violation of the law. DEA Form 222 must always be used to order drugs. Also, a practitioner ordering a controlled substance to maintain drug-dependent individuals who do not have legitimate prescriptions is in clear violation of the law. Practitioners cannot order drugs for their office using prescription pads – they must use an order form or a purchase order. Prescriptions for Schedule II drugs must be written, not faxed or called in, unless an absolute emergency exists that requires a telephone prescription order. Exceptions are made for hospices and nursing homes, however. No prescription for a Schedule II controlled substance may be refilled. Prescriptions for Schedule III or IV controlled substances may be refilled if a practitioner gives authorization. These prescriptions may not be filled or refilled more than 6 months after the date issued, nor can they be refilled more than 5 times after the date issued. After 6 months or after 5 refills, the practitioner may renew the prescription.

The advent of technology has brought "electronic prescribing" or "e-prescribing" to the forefront in order to reduce medication errors. The accuracy that e-prescribing allows for will become instrumental in reducing errors due to illegible handwriting, wrong dosing, and missed drug interactions. In e-prescribing, prescriptions are generated electronically through automated data entry and a pharmacy-linked transmission network. It features warning/alert systems, access to full medical histories, reduction of phoned-in and faxed requests, streamlined authorizations, increased patient compliance, and better reporting of the entire prescription process. Though e-prescribing is not fully in place to support controlled substance prescriptions, it is evolving into the best and most accurate form of prescribing.

FILLING PRESCRIPTIONS FOR CONTROLLED SUBSTANCES

Prescriptions for Schedule II drugs must be signed in ink, although the prescription itself can be created on a computer or handwritten. No refills are allowed; however, partial fillings are allowed only if the portion dispensed can be used in a 7-day period. After 7 days, a new prescription is needed to obtain any additional quantities. The pharmacist should notify the physician if the remaining amount is not available. Oral prescriptions are only allowed if it is an emergency. The pharmacist must identify the physician who is required to follow up with a written prescription within 72 hours. The amount dispensed for an emergency should only be that which is necessary until the written prescription can be presented. All prescriptions for controlled substances must be maintained in one of the following manners:

- A three-file system
  - One file for all Schedule II prescriptions
  - One file for all Schedule III, IV, and V prescriptions
  - One file for all other types of prescriptions
- A two-file system
  - One file for Schedule II prescriptions
  - One file for Schedules III, IV, and V prescriptions
- An alternate two-file system
  - One file for all controlled drug prescriptions
  - One file for prescription orders for all non-controlled drugs that are dispensed

LABELING OF CONTROLLED SUBSTANCES

Federal law and state statutes regulate the labeling of controlled substance prescriptions. These types of prescription orders must include the dispensing pharmacist's name and address, the pharmacy's name, the drug's serial number, and the date the prescription was filled. The prescribing physician's name, the patient's name, directions for use, and any cautionary statements must also be included. Most states have adopted laws requiring additional information to be included on the label, e.g., the telephone number of the pharmacy.

The law requires labeling of controlled substances. The containers of controlled substances must have a special symbol, printed by their manufacturer, on the label of their stock bottle designating which schedule applies. The following symbols are designed for stock bottles containing controlled substances in Schedules I through V:

CI	or	C-I
CII	or	C-II
CIII	or	C-III
CIV	or	C-IV
CV	or	C-V

The word "Schedule" does not need to be used. Each symbol must be at least twice as large as the largest letter printed on the label. If the container is too small to have a printed label, only the box and the package insert must contain the "C" symbol. Drugs in Schedules II, III, and IV must bear this label when dispensed by a pharmacy: *Federal law prohibits the transfer of this drug to any person other than the patient for whom it is prescribed.* See Figure 4-3 for an example of a controlled substance label.

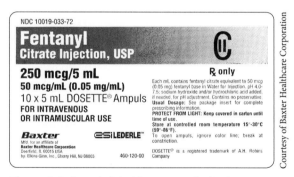

Figure 4-3 Sample label for a controlled substance.

Focus On...

Labeling Controlled Substances

These symbols are not required on prescription containers dispensed by a pharmacist to a patient in the course of his professional practice, although laws of some states may require such symbols on prescriptions dispensed to extended-care facilities.

Exemptions from Labeling Requirements – Schedule II Substances

Unit doses dispensed to an inpatient hospital or in a nursing home or other long-term care facility are exempt from prescription container labeling requirements as long as the following conditions exist:

1. A maximum of a 7-day supply may be dispensed at one time.
2. The patient does not possess the drug before he or she can use it.
3. The institution maintains appropriate security.
4. The directions for use, cautions, patient, product, and supplier are identified by the pharmacist's record-keeping system.

It is important to remember that the CSA Schedule is required on unit doses.

DISTRIBUTION

A separate DEA registration is needed for manufacturing, distributing, dispensing, or conducting research. However, a pharmacy registered to dispense a controlled substance can distribute (without being registered as a distributor) an amount of controlled substances to a physician, hospital, nursing home, or another pharmacy for general dispensing. These distributions must meet the following conditions:

1. The pharmacy or practitioner to which the controlled substance is distributed must be listed.
2. If the substance is listed in Schedules I or II, the transfer must be made with an official DEA order Form 222.
3. The distribution must be recorded as being distributed by the pharmacy and the pharmacist, or practitioner, must record the substance as being received. The pharmacy who is distributing a controlled substance must record the following information:
   - The name of the medication
   - The dosage form
   - The amount of the substance
   - The name and address of the pharmacy
   - The DEA registration number of the practitioner or the pharmacy
   - The date of distribution
4. The total number of dosage units of controlled substance distributed by a pharmacy may not exceed 5 percent of all controlled substances dispensed by the pharmacy during the 12-month period in which the pharmacy is registered. If at

any time it does exceed 5 percent, the pharmacy is required to register as a distributor as well as a pharmacy.

The DEA maintains strict controls concerning the transfer of controlled substances. If, for example, a pharmacy goes out of business, or is purchased by another company, its controlled substances may be transferred to the new owner, the supplier, the manufacturer, or a distributor that is registered to dispose of controlled substances. A pharmacy that is intending to terminate business must notify the closest DEA field office in writing prior to termination. The DEA registrant who will be receiving Schedule I or II controlled substances must issue a DEA Form 222 to the registrant who will be transferring the drugs. For Schedule III to V controlled substances, the transfer must be documented in writing, showing the drug name, dosage form, strength, quality, date transferred, and the complete names, addresses, and DEA numbers of any parties involved in the transfer.

What Would You Do?

Nicole had a back injury and was suffering from severe back pain. Her neurologist prescribed oxycodone for her. Two days later, her brother came to visit from out of state, planning to stay with Nicole for 1 week. Upon his arrival, he complained about a severe headache. Nicole gave some of the oxycodone to her brother to relieve his pain, which he then crushed up and snorted, similar to cocaine. Several days later, she found that five more oxycodone tablets were missing from her bottle. If you were Nicole, what would you do in this situation? Did she break the law?

RECORD KEEPING

Any pharmacy that handles controlled substances must keep complete and accurate records of all drugs received and dispensed. The records must be kept for 2 years. Some states require that the records must be kept for at least 5 years. Schedule II drug records must be kept separately from all other records. Any record that includes controlled substances must be made available for inspection by DEA officials. Record keeping includes: a record of inventory, a record of received drugs, and a dispersal record.

Inventory Records

The CSA requires that, every 2 years, each registrant create a complete, accurate controlled substances stock record. When the inventory of Schedule II controlled substances is done, an exact count or measure must be made. Before a new pharmacy opens, a complete inventory of all controlled substances must be made. This is known as the "initial inventory."

After opening for business, an exact count of all Schedule II substances must be made every 2 years. An estimated count of all Schedule III, IV, and V substances must also be made every 2 years, though for Schedule III and IV substances in bottles of 1,000 or greater, they must be counted exactly, not estimated. These are referred to as "biennial inventories." These records must be kept on file for at least 2 years following the date the inventory was taken.

A controlled substance "perpetual inventory" must be maintained in hospital pharmacies showing all of these substances – in retail pharmacies, it is not mandatory but is suggested. This type of inventory is designed to show how many units of each drug are actually in stock at the pharmacy.

What Would You Do?

Teresa, a pharmacy technician, was doing an initial inventory of scheduled drugs for a new pharmacy, including Schedule II drugs. She estimated the content of the scheduled drugs and recorded her estimates. When the pharmacy checked her inventory records later, he noticed that the inventory for the Schedule II drugs was not accurate. If you were Teresa, what would you have done differently?

Keeping Receipts

DEA Form 222 is used as the official form of receipt for all Schedule I and II substances. Invoices are acceptable to use as receipts for all Schedule III, IV, and V substances. Each type of receipt must have the date the item(s) were received written upon them. Controlled substances are usually clearly indicated (with red ink) on a specific page of any invoice that contains both controlled and non-controlled substances.

Receipts must contain the name and strength of each substance, dosage forms, number of dosage units, container volumes, number of received containers, and dates of receipt. The supplier's name, address, and DEA number must also be included.

Dispersal Record

Records of all drugs dispensed from the pharmacy, as well as records of all drugs removed from the pharmacy for any reason, are considered as "dispersal records." Dispersal records include DEA Form 222, invoices, record books, disposal records, and theft or loss records.

RETURNING CONTROLLED SUBSTANCES

When controlled substances from Schedule II are returned, DEA Form 222 must be used. These substances may only be returned from one DEA registrant to another. Any facility that does not have a DEA number cannot return controlled substances. All returned controlled substances must be properly labeled with product descriptions, quantities, product names, product sizes, strengths, NDC numbers, and manufacturer names.

DEALING WITH OUTDATED CONTROLLED SUBSTANCES

When controlled substances become out of date, DEA Form 41, which can be obtained online, must be used. The pharmacist must write a cover letter explaining the situation and requesting DEA permission to destroy these substances. Though these substances do not have to be destroyed by the pharmacy, they must be listed separately in their biennial inventories. Approval for destruction of these drugs is not required from the DEA if the destruction is witnessed by a Board of Pharmacy investigator. The cover letter must be attached to the completed Form 41 with signed copies of Form 41 sent to the DEA (see Figure 4-4).

Retail pharmacies may request DEA permission to destroy these substances once per year. The request must be sent to the DEA 2 weeks prior to the intended date of destruction. Two witnesses (either physicians, pharmacists, mid-level practitioners, nurses, or law enforcement officers) must witness the destruction of the substances. Many pharmacies use a product-return system wherein they may be reimbursed for part of the drug product's original cost.

THEFT OR LOSS OF CONTROLLED SUBSTANCES

The DEA office nearest the pharmacy must be notified if a controlled substance is lost or stolen. Significant losses must be reported by phone immediately. When lesser amounts are reported in writing, DEA Form 106 must be used to report this. The report must include the company's name and address, DEA number, date the theft or loss occurred, type of theft or loss, a complete list of the missing controlled substances, and the local police department's contact information, as well as an explanation of the pharmacy's container-marking system and related costs. An original copy of the report should be kept by the pharmacy, two copies should be sent to the DEA, and in most states one copy should be sent to the Board of Pharmacy. The pharmacy may also be required to send a copy to the local police department. See Figure 4-5 for an example of DEA Form 106.

OMB Approval No. 1117 - 0007	U. S. Department of Justice / Drug Enforcement Administration **REGISTRANTS INVENTORY OF DRUGS SURRENDERED**	PACKAGE NO.

The following schedule is an inventory of controlled substances which is hereby surrendered to you for proper disposition.

FROM: *(Include Name, Street, City, State and ZIP Code in space provided below.)*

Signature of applicant or authorized agent

Registrant's DEA Number

Registrant's Telephone Number

NOTE: CERTIFIED MAIL (Return Receipt Requested) IS REQUIRED FOR SHIPMENTS OF DRUGS VIA U.S. POSTAL SERVICE. See instructions on reverse (page 2) of form.

NAME OF DRUG OR PREPARATION Registrants will fill in Columns 1,2,3, and 4 ONLY.	Number of Containers	CONTENTS *(Number of grams, tablets, ounces or other units per container)*	Controlled Substance Content, *(Each Unit)*	FOR DEA USE ONLY DISPOSITION	QUANTITY GMS.	MGS.
1	2	3	4	5	6	7
1						
2						
3						
4						
5						
6						
7						
8						
9						
10						
11						
12						
13						
14						
15						
16						

FORM DEA-41 (9-01)   Previous edition dated **6-86** is usable.   *See instructions on reverse (page 2) of form.*

Figure 4-4 DEA Form 41.

DEA-41 (6/1986) Pg. 2

NAME OF DRUG OR PREPARATION Registrants will fill in Columns 1,2,3, and 4 ONLY.	Number of Containers	CONTENTS (Number of grams, tablets, ounces or other units per container)	Controlled Substance Content, (Each Unit)	FOR DEA USE ONLY		
				DISPOSITION	QUANTITY	
					GMS.	MGS.
1	*2*	*3*	*4*	*5*	*6*	*7*
17						
18						
19						
20						
21						
22						
23						
24						

The controlled substances surrendered in accordance with Title 21 of the Code of Federal Regulations, Section 1307.21, have been received in _____ packages purporting to contain the drugs listed on this inventory and have been: ** (1) Forwarded tape-sealed without opening; (2) Destroyed as indicated and the remainder forwarded tape-sealed after verifying contents; (3) Forwarded tape-sealed after verifying contents.

DATE _____   DESTROYED BY: _____

** *Strike out lines not applicable.*   WITNESSED BY: _____

INSTRUCTIONS

1. List the name of the drug in column 1, the number of containers in column 2, the size of each container in column 3, and in column 4 the controlled substance content of each unit described in column 3; e.g., morphine sulfate tabs., 3 pkgs., 100 tabs., 1/4 gr. (16 mg.) or morphine sulfate tabs., 1 pkg., 83 tabs., 1/2 gr. (32mg.), etc.

2. All packages included on a single line should be identical in name, content and controlled substance strength.

3. Prepare this form in quadruplicate. Mail two (2) copies of this form to the Special Agent in Charge, under separate cover. Enclose one additional copy in the shipment with the drugs. Retain one copy for your records. One copy will be returned to you as a receipt. No further receipt will be furnished to you unless specifically requested. Any further inquiries concerning these drugs should be addressed to the DEA District Office which serves your area.

4. There is no provision for payment for drugs surrendered. This is merely a service rendered to registrants enabling them to clear their stocks and records of unwanted items.

5. Drugs should be shipped tape-sealed via prepaid express or certified mail (**return receipt requested**) to Special Agent in Charge, Drug Enforcement Administration, of the DEA District Office which serves your area.

PRIVACY ACT INFORMATION

AUTHORITY: Section 307 of the Controlled Substances Act of 1970 (PL 91-513).
PURPOSE: To document the surrender of controlled substances which have been forwarded by registrants to DEA for disposal.
ROUTINE USES: This form is required by Federal Regulations for the surrender of unwanted Controlled Substances. Disclosures of information from this system are made to the following categories of users for the purposes stated.
  A. Other Federal law enforcement and regulatory agencies for law enforcement and regulatory purposes.
  B. State and local law enforcement and regulatory agencies for law enforcement and regulatory purposes.
EFFECT: Failure to document the surrender of unwanted Controlled Substances may result in prosecution for violation of the Controlled Substances Act.

Under the Paperwork Reduction Act, a person is not required to respond to a collection of information unless it displays a currently valid OMB control number. Public reporting burden for this collection of information is estimated to average 30 minutes per response, including the time for reviewing instructions, searching existing data sources, gathering and maintaining the data needed, and completing and reviewing the collection of information. Send comments regarding this burden estimate or any other aspect of this collection of information, including suggestions for reducing this burden, to the Drug Enforcement Administration, FOI and Records Management Section, Washington, D.C. 20537; and to the Office of Management and Budget, Paperwork Reduction Project no. 1117-0007, Washington, D.C. 20503.

Figure 4-4 DEA Form 41 *(continued)*.

REPORT OF THEFT OR LOSS OF CONTROLLED SUBSTANCES

Federal Regulations require registrants to submit a detailed report of any theft or loss of Controlled Substances to the Drug Enforcement Administration.

Complete the front and back of this form in triplicate. Forward the original and duplicate copies to the nearest DEA Office. Retain the triplicate copy for your records. Some states may also require a copy of this report.

OMB APPROVAL No. 1117-0001

1. Name and Address of Registrant (include ZIP Code)		2. Phone No. (Include Area Code)
	ZIP CODE	

3. DEA Registration Number
2 ltr. prefix   7 digit suffix

4. Date of Theft or Loss

5. Principal Business of Registrant (Check one)
1 ☐ Pharmacy   5 ☐ Distributor
2 ☐ Practitioner   6 ☐ Methadone Program
3 ☐ Manufacturer   7 ☐ Other (Specify)
4 ☐ Hospital/Clinic

6. County in which Registrant is located

7. Was Theft reported to Police?   ☐ Yes ☐ No

8. Name and Telephone Number of Police Department (Include Area Code)

9. Number of Thefts or Losses Registrant has experienced in the past 24 months

10. Type of Theft or Loss (Check one and complete items below as appropriate)
1 ☐ Night break-in   3 ☐ Employee pilferage   5 ☐ Other (Explain)
2 ☐ Armed robbery   4 ☐ Customer theft   6 ☐ Lost in transit (Complete Item 14)

11. If Armed Robbery, was anyone:
Killed? ☐ No ☐ Yes (How many)
Injured? ☐ No ☐ Yes (How many) _____

12. Purchase value to registrant of Controlled Substances taken?
$

13. Were any pharmaceuticals or merchandise taken?
☐ No ☐ Yes (Est. Value)
$

14. IF LOST IN TRANSIT, COMPLETE THE FOLLOWING:

A. Name of Common Carrier	B. Name of Consignee	C. Consignee's DEA Registration Number

D. Was the carton received by the customer? ☐ Yes ☐ No

E. If received, did it appear to be tampered with? ☐ Yes ☐ No

F. Have you experienced losses in transit from this same carrier in the past? ☐ No ☐ Yes (How Many) _____

15. What identifying marks, symbols, or price codes were on the labels of these containers that would assist in identifying the products?

16. If Official Controlled Substance Order Forms (DEA-222) were stolen, give numbers.

17. What security measures have been taken to prevent future thefts or losses?

PRIVACY ACT INFORMATION

AUTHORITY: Section 301 of the Controlled Substances Act of 1970 (PL 91-513).
PURPOSE: Report theft or loss of Controlled Substances.
ROUTINE USES: The Controlled Substances Act authorizes the production of special reports required for statistical and analytical purposes. Disclosures of information from this system are made to the following categories of users for the purposes stated:

A. Other Federal law enforcement and regulatory agencies for law enforcement and regulatory purposes.
B. State and local law enforcement and regulatory agencies for law enforcement and regulatory purposes.

EFFECT: Failure to report theft or loss of controlled substances may result in penalties under Section 402 and 403 of the Controlled Substances Act.

In accordance with the Paperwork Reduction Act of 1995, no person is required to respond to a collection of information unless it displays a ly valid OMB control number. The valid OMB control number for this collection of information is 1117-0001. Public reporting burden for this collection of information is estimated to average 30 minutes per response , including the time for reviewing instructions, searching existing data sources, gathering and maintaining the data needed, and completing and reviewing the collection of information.

FORM DEA - 106 (11-00) *Previous editions obsolete*

CONTINUE ON REVERSE

Figure 4-5 DEA Form 106.

FORM DEA-106 (Nov. 2000) Pg. 2   **LIST OF CONTROLLED SUBSTANCES LOST**

Trade Name of Substance or Preparation	Name of Controlled Substance in Preparation	Dosage Strength and Form	Quantity
Examples: Desoxyn	Methamphetamine Hydrochloride	5 mg Tablets	3 x 100
Demerol	Meperidine Hydrochloride	50 mg/ml Vial	5 x 30 ml
Robitussin A-C	Codeine Phosphate	2 mg/cc Liquid	12 Pints
1.			
2.			
3.			
4.			
5.			
6.			
7.			
8.			
9.			
10.			
11.			
12.			
13.			
14.			
15.			
16.			
17.			
18.			
19.			
20.			
21.			
22.			
23.			
24.			
25.			
26.			
27.			
28.			
29.			
30.			
31.			
32.			
33.			
34.			
35.			
36.			
37.			
38.			
39.			
40.			
41.			
42.			
43.			
44.			
45.			
46.			
47.			
48.			
49.			
50.			

I certify that the foregoing information is correct to the best of my knowledge and belief.

_____   _____   _____
Signature   Title   Date

Figure 4-5 DEA Form 106 *(continued)*.

REFILLING PRESCRIPTIONS FOR CONTROLLED SUBSTANCES

Prescriptions for a Schedule II controlled substance must not be refilled, except in certain limited circumstances. Federal law allows the partial filling of Schedule II prescriptions, and prescriptions for Schedules III or IV controlled substances may be refilled if so authorized. The DEA has published information on its Web site that discusses partial refills of Schedule III and IV substances. These are permissible as long as each partial filling is dispensed and recorded in the same manner as a refilling. The total quantity dispensed in all partial fillings cannot exceed the total quantity prescribed. No dispensing can occur after 6 months past the date of issue. Some states allow for partial refills of Schedule II drugs to ambulatory patients, often within 72 hours of the original prescription.

Focus On...

Refills

Schedule II drugs are not to be refilled. However, in certain circumstances (such as nursing homes), when individual patients need multiple, sequential prescriptions up to a 90-day supply, partial refills are allowed. There are rules for issuing multiple prescriptions on the same day for the same drug and patient. Generally, multiple prescriptions are still required. Schedule III and IV prescriptions may not be refilled more than five times after the date issued.

Recording Refills

A pharmacist, after refilling a prescription for any controlled substance in Schedules III, IV, or V, must enter (on the back of that prescription) his or her initials, the date the prescription was refilled, and the amount of drug dispensed. If they merely initial and date the back of the prescription, they shall be deemed to have dispensed a refill for the full face amount of the prescription. This initialing, dating, and adding of the amount of drug dispensed is not required if the pharmacy is using electronic data retrieval, and today, this process is used only rarely since computerization makes it unneeded.

Computerization of Refilling

A pharmacy is allowed to use a data processing system for the storage and retrieval of prescription refill information for controlled substances in Schedules III and IV. The computerized system must provide immediate retrieval of original prescription information for prescriptions that currently are authorized for refilling. The information that must be readily retrievable must include, but is not limited to: the original prescription number; date of issuance of the prescription by the practitioner; full name and address of the patient; practitioner's name and DEA registration number; the name, strength, dosage form, and quantity of the controlled substance prescribed; quantity dispensed if different from the quantity prescribed; and the total number of refills authorized by the prescriber.

In addition, the system must provide immediate retrieval of the current refill history for Schedules III and IV controlled substance prescriptions that have been authorized for refills during the past 6 months. Backup documentation (such as the daily log book or printout) can be used to show that the refill information is correct. Pharmacy technicians can help assure that this backup documentation is signed by all pharmacists who worked during the period in question. The backup documentation must be stored in a separate file at the pharmacy and maintained for a 2-year period from the dispensing date.

FACSIMILE PRESCRIPTIONS

DEA regulations permit prescriptions for Schedule II, III, IV, and V drugs to be sent via facsimile (a copy of an official document transmitted electronically via a fax machine) from the practitioner directly to the pharmacy. The pharmacist must review original, signed prescriptions for Schedule II substances. The only cases where this is not required are listed below:

- A Schedule II narcotic requiring compounding for direct parenteral or intraspinal infusion with specific instructions for a home infusion pharmacy

- A Schedule II prescription for a patient in a long-term care facility

- A Schedule II prescription for a patient in a Medicare-certified or state-certified hospice facility. The pharmacy must keep this fax for his or her records. Faxed prescriptions may also be used for hospice patients who are at home but receiving services from a certified hospice – they do not have to reside in the hospice facility.

In addition to written or oral prescribing of Schedule III, IV, and V substances, DEA regulations permit the facsimile of a written signed prescription transmitted by the prescribing practitioner or the practitioner's agent to serve as the authority for, and record of, the dispensing of a Schedule III, IV, or V substance.

Although federal DEA regulations allow for facsimile prescriptions for controlled substances, they do not authorize a practitioner to prescribe or a pharmacist to dispense controlled substances via faxed prescriptions unless *expressly provided for under the state law* in the jurisdiction in which the health care providers practice. Almost all states allow this.

STORAGE AND SECURITY REQUIREMENTS

Schedule I substances, except the very limited amounts actually being processed, must be stored in a securely locked, substantially constructed cabinet. Schedule II through V substances must also be stored as above, though pharmacies, institutional practitioners, clinical researchers, and those performing chemical analysis may disperse them throughout their non-controlled substances stock in order to obstruct theft or diversion of the controlled substances. This information can be found at http://www.deadiversion.usdoj .gov (click on "Regulations and Codified CSA"; "Code of Federal Regulations"; "Section 1301"; "Section 1301.75"). Security regulations must be stringent to prevent theft of controlled substances. All of the following help to assure strict control and security concerning controlled substances:

- An electronic alarm system
- Perimeter security
- Self-closing and locking doors
- A system of key control
- Controlled accessibility

Other security controls that affect manufacturers, distributors, shippers, and carriers include:

- The manufacturer or distributor must make a diligent effort to determine that persons ordering from them are also registered themselves.
- The distributor must develop and maintain a system for detecting "suspicious orders" and reporting them.
- The distributor must report all losses of controlled substances, including goods lost in transit, to the DEA on Form

106, even if the substances are recovered. It is *the responsibility of the shipper, not the carrier,* to report such losses.

• The registrant is responsible for selecting a reputable and secure warehouse for storage as well as a reputable and security-conscious carrier to transport controlled substances.

Focus On...

Storage and Security

Various states allow pharmacy technicians to have access to the safe where scheduled drugs are stored, under direct observation of the pharmacist, and can conduct controlled substance inventories. They must keep in mind that the safe must be always locked when not in use — security of Schedule II drugs is of primary importance. Only the pharmacist is allowed to unlock and open the safe.

DEA INSPECTIONS

The Controlled Substances Act specifically requires an administrative search warrant for most nonconsensual DEA inspections. Therefore, for an agent of the DEA to enter any DEA-registered premises, the agent must state the purpose for the inspection and present appropriate identification. In addition, the agent must obtain an informed consent from the registrant, secure an administrative inspection warrant, or fit into one of the special exceptions set forth in the state statutes. The act recognizes certain circumstances in which an inspection warrant is not required, such as the initial registration inspection, inspection of mobile vehicles, emergencies, or dangerous health situations. Pharmacy technicians should be aware that they should immediately refer any DEA agents to the pharmacist in charge.

SUMMARY

The Comprehensive Drug Abuse Prevention and Control Act of 1970 is called the Controlled Substances Act (CSA). This law is enforced with the Drug Enforcement Administration (DEA). Under the jurisdiction of the CSA, drugs with potential for abuse are classified into five Schedules: I, II, III, IV, and V.

Schedule I agents have a high potential for abuse and no accepted medical use in the United States (except for the recent approval for medical marijuana in relation to specific, approved conditions). Schedule V agents have the lowest abuse potential of the controlled substances and consist of preparations containing limited quantities of certain narcotic drugs.

Pharmacies that deal with manufacturing, dispensing, or distributing any controlled substances are obligated to register with the DEA unless they are exempted. No prescription for Schedule II controlled substances may be refilled. Schedule III or IV controlled substances may be refilled if a practitioner gives authorization. These prescriptions may not be filled or refilled more than 6 months after the date issued, nor can they be refilled more than 5 times after the date issued. However, there is no federal limit on how long prescriptions are valid. Pharmacy technicians must understand the complete concepts of the laws that relate to controlled substances. They also must be familiar with regulations and registration concerning controlled substances, filling prescriptions, labeling, record keeping, inventory records, and the role of the DEA.

SETTING THE SCENE

The following discussion and responses relate to the opening "Setting the Scene" scenario:

- Anthony cannot sign Form 222 to order Schedule II drugs because he does not have Power of Attorney permitting him to do so.

- Anthony should know, after 10 years of work, that he cannot sign this form without Power of Attorney; he will most likely be verbally reprimanded, but it is possible that he could lose his job in this situation.

- The DEA only allows specific licensed pharmacists and those with Power of Attorney to order Schedule II drugs and sign the Form 222 which is used to do so.

REVIEW QUESTIONS

Multiple Choice

1. Schedule I drugs:

    A.   have currently accepted medical use
    B.   have a low potential for abuse
    C.   have a high potential for abuse
    D.   include drugs such as methadone

2. The drugs with the highest potential for abuse, having a currently accepted medical use in the United States, are classified as which of the following Schedules?

     A. I
     B. II
     C. IV
     D. V

3. Which of the following agencies oversees controlled substances and recommends prosecution for individuals who illegally distribute them?

     A. FDA
     B. CDC
     C. HIPAA
     D. DEA

4. Anabolic steroids are classified in which of the following Schedules?

     A. II
     B. III
     C. IV
     D. V

5. Diphenoxylate (with atropine) is listed in which of the following Schedules?

     A. I
     B. II
     C. IV
     D. V

6. Which of the following drugs is classified in Schedule IV?

     A. diphenoxylate
     B. anabolic steroids
     C. methadone
     D. benzodiazepines

7. Drugs in Schedules II, III, and IV must bear which of the following statements?

     A. Federal law prohibits the transfer of this drug to any person other than the patient for whom it was prescribed
     B. Federal law allows partial refilling
     C. May refill up to 10 times
     D. May refill up to 5 times

8. Significant losses of controlled substances must be reported:

   A. in writing to the DEA within 7 days
   B. in writing to the DEA within 72 hours
   C. immediately, by phone, to the nearest DEA office
   D. none of the above

9. Which of the following statements is not true regarding the maintenance of files for Schedule drugs?

   A. one file is used for Schedule II drugs dispensed
   B. one file is used for Schedule III, IV, and V drugs dispensed
   C. one file is used for Schedule I and II drugs dispensed
   D. one file is used for prescription orders for all other drugs

10. Schedule II substances do not have to be labeled according to standard labeling requirements if:

    A. they are unit doses dispensed in a nursing home
    B. they are unit doses dispensed for elderly patients
    C. they are unit doses dispensed for pregnant women
    D. they are unit doses dispensed for newborn babies in hospitals

11. The CSA requires each DEA registrant to create a complete controlled substances stock record:

    A. every 2 years
    B. every year
    C. every 3 years
    D. every 5 years

12. In most types of pharmacy practice, controlled substances should be kept in a:

    A. locked cabinet
    B. refrigerator
    C. laminaire airflow hood
    D. freezer

13. The total number of dosage units of controlled substances distributed by a pharmacy to another registrant during a 12-month period should not exceed:

    A. 1 percent of their total amount
    B. 5 percent of their total amount
    C. 10 percent of their total amount
    D. 15 percent of their total amount

14. In most states, pharmacists are usually given certificates of registration which are granted for a period of:

    A. 10 to 12 years
    B. 10 to 12 months
    C. 1 to 3 years
    D. 3 to 5 years

15. Schedule III and IV prescriptions may not be refilled more than:

    A. 1 time
    B. 2 times
    C. 3 times
    D. 5 times

Fill in the Blank

1. Controlled substances have been categorized according to their potential for _____ and their _____ abilities.

2. Amphetamines and codeine are usually classified in _____.

3. Acetaminophen with codeine, and hydrocodone with APAP, are examples of _____.

4. Diphenoxylate hydrochloride with atropine sulfate (Lomotil) is a Schedule V preparation that requires a _____.

5. Controlled substances from Schedule II are ordered by submitting DEA Form _____.

6. The total number of dosage units of controlled substances distributed to other registrants by a pharmacy may not exceed _____ of all controlled substances dispensed by the pharmacy during a _____-month period.

7. Inventory records for Schedule II drugs must be kept on file for at least _____ years following the date the inventory was taken.

8. Though not required, controlled substances are often marked with red ink on any invoice that contains both controlled and _____ substances.

9. For destroying controlled substances, DEA Form _____ must be used.

10. When controlled substances are stolen or lost, DEA Form _____ must be used.

CASE STUDY

Jackie is a pharmacy technician. She receives a faxed prescription for a Schedule II drug for a patient in a long-term care facility. She questions her supervisor about the prescription. Robert, her supervisor, asks her, "Do you think that our state allows us to fill a faxed prescription for Schedule II drugs?" John, another pharmacy staff member, overhears this and says "Yes, we are okay. DEA regulations permit faxed prescriptions of Schedule II drugs for patients in long-term care facilities." "Maybe so," Robert says, "but I still want to know her response, because I do not know what state law says." John replies, "It doesn't matter; the DEA is a federal agency. Federal law overrides state law. Go ahead and fill it, Jackie, you will be all right." Robert disagrees, saying, "I don't think we can make that assumption."

1. Without knowing anything else about this case, who do you think is correct?

2. What else could Robert, Jackie, and John have done to verify the correct information?

3. What agency would regulate Schedule II prescriptions in their state?

RELATED INTERNET SITES

Use the following key words to search for additional information at these sites: "controlled substances act," "controlled substances," "Schedule II drugs," "DEA."

http://www.deadiversion.usdoj.org

http://www.deadiversion.usdoj.gov; **click on "Regulations and Codified CSA"; "Code of Federal Regulations"; "Section 1301"; "Section 1301.75"**

http://www.deadiversion.usdoj.gov; **click on "Publications"; "Manuals"; "Pharmacist's Manual"**

http://www.deaecom.gov

http://www.dealookup.com

http://www.fda.gov

http://www.fda.gov/search/databases.html

http://www.napra.org

http://www.nccusl.org

http://www.ntis.gov

http://www.painandthelaw.org

http://www.purdue.edu

http://www.usdoj.gov

REFERENCES

Abood, R. (2005). *Pharmacy Practice and the Law* (4th ed.). Jones and Bartlett.

Fink, J. L., Vivian, J. C., & Bernstein, I. B. (2006). *Pharmacy Law Digest* (40th ed.). Wolters Kluwer Health.

Fred, L. Y. (2005). *Manual for Pharmacy Technicians* (3rd ed.). ASHP.

Mizner, J. J. (2006). *Mosby's Review for the PTCB Certification Examination.* Mosby/Elsevier.

Reiss, B. S., & Hall, G. D. (2006). *Guide to Federal Pharmacy Law* (5th ed.). Apothecary Press.

The Health Insurance Portability and Accountability Act (HIPAA)

OBJECTIVES

Upon completion of this chapter, the reader should be able to:

1. Explain how the HIPAA Privacy Rule benefits the pharmacy and patients.
2. Identify the difference between Title I and Title II of HIPAA.
3. List the rights that patients have under the Privacy Rule.
4. Explain what is expected of pharmacy technicians in relation to the Privacy Rule.
5. Describe how to protect patient confidentiality.
6. Explain why a technician cannot discuss protected health information with a patient's friends and family.
7. Discuss the general purpose of the HIPAA-mandated administrative code sets.
8. State the purpose of the HIPAA Electronic Health Care Transactions and Code Sets standards.
9. Describe the purpose of the Office of the Inspector General.
10. Compare fraud and abuse.

KEY TERMS

Compliance program guidelines – HIPAA-related privacy, training, and security regulations designed to focus on, correct, and maintain good health-care practices.

Disclosure – Transferring information, releasing information, providing access to information, or divulging information in any manner.

Electronic data interchange (EDI) – A set of standards for structuring electronic information intended to be exchanged between different entities.

Electronic medical records (EMR) – Preferred method of record storage (over paper records) because their electronic format can be accessed more quickly and takes less room to store.

Encryption – Transforming information via an algorithm to make it unreadable to anyone who does not possess the decryption information required to read it.

Extranet – A private network that uses Internet protocols, network connections, and sometimes telecommunication devices to share information with outside entities.

Medical code sets – Sets of alphanumeric codes used for encoding medical conditions, diseases, procedures, and other information.

Notice of Privacy Practices (NOPP) – A document that explains to patients how his or her PHI may be used and disclosed.

Office of the Inspector General (OIG) – Governmental office that investigates various organizations, including health-care organizations, to assure integrity and efficiency in their operations.

Protected health information (PHI) – All stored health information that relates to a past, present, or future physical or mental health condition.

Security Rule – A HIPAA-related regulation that specifies how PHI is protected on computer networks, the Internet, the extranet, and disks and other storage media.

Treatment, payment, and health care operations (TPHCO) – This concerns PHI that may be shared in order to provide treatment, process payment, and operate the medical business.

SETTING THE SCENE

Katie, a pharmacy technician with 15 years of experience, works for an institutional pharmacy. Her sister is a nurse, and her brother is a cardiovascular technician. Katie's mother-in-law has been a nurse for 40 years, and she has worked for a local internist for more than 25 years. At a family picnic, Katie's mother-in-law asked Katie if she was aware that their neighbor Joe had been diagnosed with HIV and syphilis. Katie asked her how she knew this, and her mother-in-law told her that Joe had been in the medical office where she worked, and she had looked at his lab results in his medical record. Katie told her husband about Joe's condition, and at their next golf game, he told Joe he was so sorry to hear about his diagnosis. Joe was angry, and asked how he knew about this.

Critical Thinking

- What should Katie and her relatives have done?

- How could their discussion of Joe's private health information jeopardize their careers?

OVERVIEW

The creation of privacy and security laws was aimed at more efficient pharmacy practice and faster reimbursement. The advent of technology has increased the practice of and efficiencies of pharmacy. However, electronic records and processing of data lead to concerns related to maintaining the privacy of patients. HIPAA laws were put into place to standardize controls over the dissemination of private health records. Many health-care professionals feel that they can't discuss anything about any patient at all – no matter where they are or when the topic arises. If pharmacy technicians understand HIPAA compliances, they can feel secure in dealing with patients and other individuals in the pharmacy.

THE GOAL OF HIPAA

The primary goals of the Health Insurance Portability and Accountability Act include improving the portability (ability to transmit and transfer information) and continuity of health-care coverage. It affects both groups and individuals, and is intended to reduce abuse, fraud, and waste in health-care delivery and insurance. HIPAA strives to promote the use of medical savings accounts, improve access to long-term health-care coverage and services, and simplify health insurance administration.

Under HIPAA, health-care providers ensure that patient confidentiality is always maintained. The use and disclosure of **protected health information (PHI)** by covered entities is controlled by HIPAA. PHI must be identified to be protected and it is important to understand that all health information (whether verbal, written, or electronic) should be protected. Patients have the right to be told how their PHI can be used. HIPAA allows employees to take their health coverage with them when they change jobs. It allows patients to have better access to their own health information while controlling how others can access it. HIPAA consists of two parts. Title I focuses on continuation of health insurance coverage. Title II controls the private health information of individuals.

Title I: Health Insurance Reform

Before HIPAA, people who had private health insurance did not have as many rights as did people who were covered by Medicare or Medicaid. Most private insurance comes from employers, individual health-care plans, or from the Federal Employees' Health Benefits Program. State law regulates many types of health insurance, though employer-offered health plans are regulated by the Employee Retirement Income and Security Act of 1974 (ERISA).

The Consolidated Omnibus Budget Reconciliation Act of 1985 (COBRA) allows employees who are leaving a job to elect to continue their previous employer's health coverage for a limited time. Under COBRA, employees must pay the premium for their coverage themselves, and it is usually higher than what they were paying when still employed at their previous job. COBRA was modified by Title I of HIPAA, with exclusions for pre-existing health conditions being limited. Title I also gave certain people the ability to enroll into new health-care plans of different types.

Title II: Administrative Simplification

Title II of HIPAA restricted electronic transferring of health-care data, allowed patients more rights to their own personal health information, and put in place better security of this information. Due to rising costs, Title II sought to reduce paperwork, simplify Internet form processing, and standardize the administration of health-care information.

The use of electronic data interchange (EDI) was encouraged to exchange routine business information between computers. Title II of HIPAA promoted the establishment of national electronic health-care transaction standards. It established national identifiers for health-care providers, employers, and even health insurance plans. The five basic provisions of HIPAA Title II are as follows:

- Electronic health information transaction standards – this includes health-care benefits coordination, claims, eligibility, enrollment, payment, and security

- Penalties – this assigned fines and imprisonment to specific violations

- Privacy – this gave Health and Human Services the task of establishing health information standards, and the ability to set privacy regulations if Congress did not put privacy legislation into place

- Provider and health plan mandate and timetable – this allowed 2 years for providers and health plans to start using the new HIPAA standards

- State law preemption – this allowed HIPAA to supersede state laws unless Health and Human Services decided otherwise; however, when a state law is stronger, it must be followed

COMPLYING WITH HIPAA

Those who must comply with HIPAA are referred to as "covered entities" (CEs). These entities provide health-care services regularly, and send HIPAA-protected information electronically. HIPAA governs three types of covered entities: clearinghouses (claims handlers and companies that manage electronic medical records), health insurance plans, and health-care providers. State laws that relate to HIPAA should be followed because they may be more stringent than the actual related HIPAA requirements. A state law is more stringent when it:

- Grants better access rights to a patient's own protected health information (PHI)

- Prohibits a use or disclosure of PHI that a HIPAA regulation would allow

- Provides more information that can be disclosed to an individual upon request

- Requires record keeping of greater detail

- Requires more focused, limited, or narrowed authorization

Health insurance plans include group health plans, health maintenance organizations (HMOs), Medicare, Medicaid, supplemental Medicare policies, long-term policies, employee benefit plans, TRICARE, CHAMPVA, the Indian Health Service, the Federal Employees Health Benefits Program, approved child health plans, high-risk plans, and others. Health-care providers include hospitals, nursing facilities, rehabilitation facilities, hospices, home health care, pharmacies, private practices, dental practices, labs, chiropractors, osteopaths, podiatrists, and therapists.

Direct providers are those that provide direct treatment to patients. Indirect providers include labs that handle patient test results. HIPAA also works with business associates (BA) that relate to health care, including: accreditation agencies, accountants, information technology (IT) contractors, lawyers, medical transcription services, coding services, collection agents, third-party claimants, and independent contractors.

PRIVACY STANDARDS

Pharmacies have increased controls over the way they manage and store patient information. This is a result of the Privacy Rule of 2003. Patients have a right to confidentiality and the protection of their protected health information (PHI). Under the HIPAA Privacy Rule, this information belongs to patients, and they have the right to control who is able to view it. However, health-care providers who create medical records about patients also have some legal claim as to how these records are used. Access to medical records must be protected by health-care personnel, including pharmacy technicians, who must know which types of information they can release.

Discarded patient information (DPI) must be handled with great care. When patient records (either electronic or paper) are to be discarded, they should be destroyed by a licensed, bonded company. Computer storage media containing patient records must be completely wiped (erased) of all data so that no trace of patient information may remain. It is not sufficient to simply delete patient files because computer hard drives, among other storage media devices, retain files in various forms even though they may no longer appear in the file directories. DPI must never be thrown into the trash because documented cases exist of individuals who have stolen both paper records and computer disks containing hundreds or thousands of patient records. From these, thieves may obtain social security numbers, account information, and more. Identity theft is rampant in today's society, and the proper methods of discarding patient information must be undertaken.

Focus On...

Protected Health Information

PHI is health information that relates to a past, present, or future physical or mental health condition.

The Medical Record

Medical records contain information about a patient's health over time. They are shared among the health-care professionals who need them to provide accurate patient care. The medical record documents all the medical history of a patient in chronological order. The medical standards of care (in each state) ensure that every patient receives the best quality care that they are guaranteed. Since medical records are legal documents, their accuracy is vital in documenting that appropriate medical care has been given to each patient. Visits to health-care providers are documented thoroughly, and the same form of documentation is undertaken for every visit (also known as an "encounter"). Aside from the patient's name, the other information that is documented for each encounter is the date and reason for the visit, related medical history, physical exam, review of medications, review of tests, diagnosis, review of procedures and treatments, care plan, advice that was given to the patient, and the health-care professional's signature.

More health-care providers are using electronic medical records today, and paper records are becoming rarer. Electronic medical records (EMR) are preferred over paper records because they can be accessed more quickly, and take less room to store. They also may be shared between authorized health-care professionals more easily than paper records can. *Electronic health records*, which are often confused with electronic medical records, are actually not the same at all. An EHR relies on an EMR being in place. An EMR is the legal record of a care delivery organization upon which an EHR is based. An EMR is owned by the care delivery organization, while an EHR is owned by the patient or person who has a stake in the outcome. An EMR is not really interactive with the patient, while an EHR provides interactive patient access.

Protected Health Information

HIPAA privacy standards were established in 2003 to protect personal health information. These standards require that privacy policies must be appropriate to the services provided, and a specific person within the organization must oversee them. Patients' records must always be protected by trained employees who understand the legal regulations about who may have access to them. Patients must be told how their protected health information (PHI) can be used, and by whom. Protected health information is defined as the stored information about a patient. This information can be transmitted electronically, via the Internet and other methods. It includes all of a patient's basic information as well as that of relatives, employers, and health insurance providers.

Often, a pharmacy has a designated privacy and security officer who handles disclosure of PHI. This officer usually receives referred requests from patients to access or amend their records, and strives to handle them in a timely manner.

Only the minimum amount of PHI should be disclosed in any situation. This *minimum necessary standard* protects against too much information being given to any specific person or entity. A group of medical records is known as a *designated record set (DRS)*, including a provider's medical and billing records. Insurance companies include other information in their designated record sets such as payments and claims. Providers must establish a *Notice of Privacy Practices (NOPP)*, which details their policies and procedures, and make these documents available to anyone who requests them. It is required that patients sign an additional document stating that they have read and reviewed the provider's NOPP.

Focus On...

Protected Health Information

When a patient requests that his or her health information not be disclosed to anyone, the health-care provider must follow through on this request. Example: A woman requested that her PHI not be disclosed to anyone. Soon after, her husband, who was in the process of divorcing her, asked for her PHI from their pharmacy because he said he needed it for tax purposes. A young attendant gave him the information, which he proceeded to use in court against his wife to prove that she was taking prescribed drugs that impaired her judgment and ability to function normally. Her PHI should not have been given to him under any circumstances since she had requested no disclosure.

Protected health information includes the following:

- *Patient name*
- *Patient addresses*
- *All dates relating to the patient's age and medical history*
- *Phone numbers, fax numbers, e-mail addresses, and Web site addresses*
- *Social security number*
- *Medical record numbers*
- *Health plan beneficiary numbers*
- *Various account numbers*
- *Certificate and license numbers*
- *Vehicle identification and related numbers*
- *Medical device identifiers and serial numbers*
- *Fingerprints, voiceprints, and other biometric identifiers*
- *Photographs of the patient's face and any other identifying photographs*
- *Other identifying numbers, codes, or characteristics*

Focus On...

Confidentiality

In general, the patient's ethical right to confidentiality and privacy is protected by law. Only the patient can waive this right regarding his or her own health information.

Disclosure of Protected Health Information

Disclosure occurs when the entity holding the information performs any of the following actions causing the information to move outside the entity:

- Releasing

- Transferring

- Providing access

- Divulging (in any manner)

PHI may be used or disclosed by providers as long as the use or disclosure relates to treatment, payment, and the operation of the provider's business activities. Treatment, payment, and health care operations are referred to as "TPHCO". As related to PHI, treatment mostly concerns discussions with other health-care providers. Payment refers mostly to health insurance, while "health-care operations" includes training and accreditation. Providers are allowed to share information while conducting normal business activities, such as quality improvement. The release of PHI to any outside entity is referred to as *disclosure*. Disclosure may be made by e-mail, fax, orally, or in writing. If the use of patient information does not fall under TPHCO, written authorization must be obtained before the information can be shared with anyone.

People who are acting on the behalf of a patient, such as family members and others, may receive certain PHI. Usually, the patient is simply asked if the release of the specific information is okay with them. Providers must be very careful when deciding if a person is allowed to have the PHI of any patient. For children, the parents' or guardians' approval should be obtained before disclosing the child's PHI. However, in some cases, a child must give permission for their records to be disclosed. Children's access to their own records is governed by state law. In recent years, many new laws have been enacted that protect the disclosure of the PHI of emancipated, married, pregnant, and other minors – even to their parents. It is a good idea for pharmacy technicians to refer issues related to the disclosure of a child's PHI to the pharmacist or privacy officer.

Certain disclosure always requires the patient's approval. This usually means the patient will have to sign an authorization form. For example, insurance companies sometimes require medical history of drug use, mental disorders, and sexually transmitted diseases. Providers must have written authorization from the patient in order to share this type of information with insurance companies.

Judicial orders can override a patient's approval for the release of their PHI. Subpoenas for court appearances and testimony have strong authority over disclosure of PHI. In addition, PHI may be released to researchers who are studying patient data for clinical reasons. State and federal prisoners have less protection concerning the disclosure of their PHI, though state statutes may overrule

HIPAA in certain circumstances. In-depth PHI about a patient's psychotherapy cannot be disclosed in most cases. However, national security entities may have access to PHI generally any time they request it.

Focus On...

Disclosure

Information is disclosed when it is transmitted between or among organizations.

Patients' Rights

Patients have the right to view and copy their PHI with 30 days of request, either free or for a reasonable fee as per HIPAA regulations. They can request amendments (changes) to any incorrect parts of their PHI, and these must usually be completed within 30 days. Patients may request an "accounting of disclosures," though many disclosures (such as those made for TPHCO) do not have to be included in what the patient is shown. Patients can also ask for confidential communications that use different addresses, phone numbers, email addresses, etc., than are listed in their medical record. Complaints against providers' handling of PHI may be made to the Office for Civil Rights (OCR). Additionally, certain restrictions against uses or disclosures of PHI may be requested. Many states have more stringent rules, as well as shorter time limits for responses to requests.

You Be the Judge

Mr. Pelosi was admitted to Pharrish Medical Center for the treatment of a sexually transmitted disease. A pharmacy technician who had access to his chart did not comply with the HIPAA Privacy Rule, and joked with a hospital janitor about Mr. Pelosi's condition. Later, the janitor, working in Mr. Pelosi's hospital room, told Mr. Pelosi not to worry, because he himself had had the same condition at one time, and that the hospital would take good care of him. Mr. Pelosi asked him how he knew about his condition, and the janitor mentioned the pharmacy technician who told him. Infuriated at this breach of his privacy, Mr. Pelosi called his lawyer and told him to file a lawsuit against the technician. In your judgment, can Mr. Pelosi sue the technician?

Patient Notification

The HIPAA Privacy Rule changed the way patients are informed about the HIPAA compliance of covered entities. Using the Notice of Privacy Practices (NOPP), providers explain to patients how their PHI may be used and disclosed. These NOPPs discuss patient access to their own information, patient rights in full, and how to register complaints. These notices explain how the covered entity operates, and give points of contact for patients who need help concerning their PHI, as well as when the NOPP became effective for each patient. An NOPP also covers how the covered entity gets authorization regarding the use and disclosure of PHI. It explains that patients must sign and date authorization forms giving specific entities access to their PHI. Patients must sign an acknowledgement of the receipt of an NOPP or record an explanation if it cannot be obtained.

SECURITY STANDARDS

The HIPAA security standards describe how electronic PHI must be safeguarded. It is important to understand these security standards. All health-care professionals participate in the protection of patient's records.

Focus On...

Physical Safeguards

Physical safeguards are security measures designed to protect a covered entity's electronic information system. They relate to the protection of buildings and equipment from natural and environmental hazards and unauthorized intrusion.

HIPAA Security

HIPAA security standards focus on electronic PHI, not those records that are kept on paper. Electronic protected health information is also referred to as "ePHI". These records may be stored in computers and related peripheral devices, and transmitted over computer networks, the Internet, and removable media that interfaces with computers.

The goals of ePHI include availability, confidentiality, and integrity of the information included within. Covered entities must use *risk analysis* to determine potential security threats to ePHI. They must then manage these risks with policies and procedures designed to protect against them. Security risks that may threaten ePHI include computer system changes, identity theft, malware (harmful computer programs), natural disasters, power outages, and subversive threats. Computer systems and networks should have security measures implemented to protect them from threats that occur from outside or within the organization.

In February 2003, final regulations were issued regarding the administrative, physical, and technical safeguards that protect the HIPAA-regulated health information, and its confidentiality, integrity, and availability. The Security Rule specifies how patient information is protected on computer networks, the Internet, the extranet, and disks and other storage media.

Focus On...

HIPAA Training

Federal law requires that all workers, of all covered entities, be trained on the policies and procedures for the protection of the confidentiality, integrity, and security of individually identifiable health information.

Mobile Devices and Media

Devices that are termed "mobile" or "portable" include backup media, home computers, laptop computers, memory cards, personal digital assistants (PDAs), public workstations, remote access devices, smart phones, USB flash drives, and wireless access points. HIPAA has established further guidelines known as the *HIPAA Security Guidance for Remote Use of and Access to Electronic Protected Health Information.* These guidelines focus on the off-site use of ePHI. They advise covered entities to limit all forms of remote access, use encryption and virus protection, and back up all ePHI that is used by remote systems.

Faxes and E-mail

HIPAA also requires protection of PHI when using faxes and e-mail. People on the receiving end of these communications may be unauthorized to view the contents, but may have the opportunity to see them regardless. HIPAA suggests that all fax numbers and e-mail addresses be verified before transmission. In addition, HIPAA recommends the inclusion of a "confidentiality notice" instructing that whoever receives the communication in error should immediately contact the sender and destroy the information received. Fax machines should require security mechanisms in order to operate them – this can greatly reduce the amount of compromised PHI.

Focus On...

Faxes and E-mail

A drug manufacturer accidentally revealed its entire patient e-mail address list when sending out promotional e-mails to its customers – since the drug in question was an antidepressant, this inadvertent publication of private health information could have disastrous consequences affecting these patients' employment, families, and more. Faxes and e-mails of PHI are dangerous because of the possibility of someone else on the receiving end seeing this information.

HIPAA TRANSACTIONS

HIPAA has set forth requirements concerning electronic data interchange (EDI) to simplify administration information exchange. Health-care professionals should understand the related code sets and national identifiers (such as social security numbers and numbers derived from them) used in these transactions.

HIPAA Electronic Health-Care Transactions

All providers are required by HIPAA to use the same code sets, identifiers, and transaction when health-care information is transmitted. These include claims, claim status, encounter information, inquiries, and payment or remittance advice. These standards are known as *The HIPAA Electronic Health Care Transactions and Code Sets (TCS)*.

Transaction Standards

HIPAA requires that transfers of ePHI for specific business purposes must comply with specific transaction standards. These standards apply to all methods of electronic transmission, including special "extranet" links to authorized connected parties, the Internet, leased or dial-up lines, networks, or on mobile storage media. HIPAA transactions are divided into areas of medical business as follows: benefits, claims and equivalent encounters, claim status, eligibility inquires, enrollment/disenrollment, payments and remittance, referrals, and more.

The National Council for Prescription Drug Programs (NCPDP) creates and promotes data transfer standards as they relate to the practice of pharmacy. Members of the NCPDP may receive education tailored to their pharmacy practice, and also receive database services. The NCPDP standards focus on diverse areas of pharmacy practice, including: telecommunication, product identification, standard identifiers, manufacturer rebates, government programs, professional pharmacy services, electronic prescribing, long-term care, safety concerns, insurance, and more. As it relates to HIPAA, the NCPDP has subsections that focus on: the National Provider ID (NPI), the Strategic National Implementation Process, HIPAA transactions and code sets, privacy, enforcement, security, employer IDs, and Designated Standard Maintenance Organizations (DSMOs).

Medical Code Sets

Medical code sets are used to encode data elements concerning specific diagnoses and clinical procedures. Alphanumeric codes are used. Diseases, procedures, supplies, treatments, and other data have unique codes. There are six code sets used for clinical information. These include:

- ICD-9-CM (for identifying diseases and conditions)
- HCPCS (for items, supplies, and non-physician services)
- CPT-4 (for medical procedures and services)
- ICD Volume 3 codes (for inpatient hospital services)
- NDC (for drug products)
- CDT-4 (for dental services)

The ICD-9 codes were developed as part of the *International Classification of Diseases, Ninth Revision, Clinical Modification (ICD-9-CM)*.

Administrative Code Sets

Non-medical code sets are also known as "administrative code sets." These are used for administrative information, and include simple and complex codes. For example, simple codes include abbreviations for states and locations. Complex codes may refer to payments, claims, providers, and places of service.

HIPAA ENFORCEMENT

The HIPAA Security Rule requires that covered entities implement policies and procedures that will prevent, detect, contain, and correct security violations. HIPAA enforces its standards and regulations, as well as abuse and fraud that relates to them. Health-care professionals should understand HIPAA regulations and penalties thoroughly. They should know HIPAA's suggestions and steps to avoid improper conduct. The HIPAA "final enforcement rule" of 2006 clarified that acts that are committed, as well as omissions (failures to complete HIPAA-required acts), are both violations.

HIPAA Enforcement Agencies

Various government agencies enforce HIPAA. The Department of Justice (DOJ) prosecutes criminal violations. The Centers for Medicare and Medicaid Services (CMS) enforce non-privacy standards, the Electronic Health Care Transaction and Code Set Rule (TCS), the National Employer Identifier Number Rule (EIN), the Security Rule, and rules that relate to national identifiers. The Office for Civil Rights (OCR) enforces civil violations of HIPAA privacy standards. The Office of Inspector General (OIG) prosecutes fraud and abuse in the health industry while overseeing Medicare and Medicaid.

Fraud and Abuse Regulation

Health-care fraud and abuse may harm patients financially and even in medical terms, if unsafe procedures are performed as a result. The *Health Care Fraud and Abuse Control Program* enforces HIPAA regulations and government standards, working with the Office of Inspector General and the Department of Justice. The *False Claims Act* prohibits false claims or misrepresentations, and rewards "whistle-blowers" who alert them to cases of fraud. Other regulations focus on "kickbacks" (incentives given to those who defraud others), "self-referrals" (referring patients to an entity in which the referrer receives some monetary compensation), and fraud compliance education.

The Compliance Plan

Compliance plans are designed to avoid illegal practices. Many health-care providers create compliance plans to stay in line with government regulations, develop consistent policies and procedures, train their staff, and eliminate errors. Compliance plans also serve as legal defense in the case of prosecution for fraud. The Office of the Inspector General (OIG) has created compliance program guidelines for many areas of health care, including: pharmacies, laboratories, home health agencies, medical billing companies, nursing facilities, private practices, hospitals, and manufacturers.

Compliance plans should contain written policies and procedures, appointments of officers and a committee, auditing/monitoring measures, communication measures, systems of discipline, error correction methods, and employee training methods. "Codes of conduct" should be established in order to comply with government regulations, maintain accurate records, and provide high-quality and ethical patient care. Internal audits should be conducted regularly to assure that the compliance plan is being followed.

Violations and Penalties

All health-care employees who deal with PHI must comply with HIPAA. Ethical or legal breaches of confidentiality may result in many different penalties, including fines, termination, and imprisonment. Criminal penalties, which are usually assessed for intentional misuse of PHI, can be as high as $250,000 in fines and up to 10 years in prison. These types of penalties are given for knowing misuse of PHI, misuse involving false pretenses, and profiting from misuse of PHI that causes malicious harm. Civil penalties can be as high as

$25,000 in fines per year if repeated violations occur. These types of penalties are given for violating privacy on an unintentional basis.

Examples of recently reported violations of HIPAA disclosure regulations include:

- Publishing a woman's PHI online regarding an abortion – this action resulted in her being harassed by an anti-abortion group; she successfully sued the hospital who published the information

- A man was automatically enrolled in a "depression" counseling program by his employer after his medical records were released to them from his drug management company; he had taken anti-depressants previously but was no longer in need of them

- A famous entertainer's PHI was released to her manager; later, after the two ceased their working relationship, he published her records to a national tabloid

SUMMARY

The primary goals of HIPAA include improving the portability and continuity of health-care coverage. It also attempts to improve access to long-term health-care coverage and services, promote the use of medical savings accounts, and simplify health insurance administration.

HIPAA is made up of two parts. Title I focuses on continuation of health insurance coverage, while Title II controls private health information for individuals. Title II also restricts electronic transfer of health-care data, allows patients more rights concerning their protected health information (PHI), and improves security measures for this information.

HIPAA regulates clearinghouses, health-care providers, and health insurance plans. In 2003, the Privacy Rule was established, which changed the ways that pharmacies stored and managed PHI. This basically means that it changed the way pharmacies transmitted information to insurance companies.

Patients have a right to confidentiality as well as protection of their PHI. Disclosure (the release of PHI to any outside entity) can be done by e-mail, by fax, orally, or in writing. If the use of PHI does not focus on treatment, payment, and operations (TPHCO), then written authorization must be obtained before it can be shared.

Patients also have the right to examine and copy their PHI within 30 days of requesting to do so. HIPAA's 30 day rule is longer than the similar rules of many states. They can do this for free or for a small fee, as described in HIPAA. The security standards set forth by HIPAA are mostly concerned with electronic PHI, not records kept on paper. The goals of using electronic PHI include better availability, stricter confidentiality, and preserved integrity of the information. To assure that timelines are met, prompt referral to the privacy officer is critical.

SETTING THE SCENE

The following discussion and responses relate to the opening "Setting the Scene" scenario:

- Katie and her mother-in-law must not discuss private health information of any patient as this does not respect the privacy and confidentiality of the patient.

- According to the Privacy Rule of 2003, patients have a right to confidentiality and the protection of their private health information.

REVIEW QUESTIONS

Multiple Choice

1. Title II of HIPAA is referred to as which of the following?

   A. COBRA
   B. NPPM
   C. Administrative Simplification
   D. Health Insurance reform

2. Hospitals, pharmacists, physicians, and therapists are examples of:

   A. business associates
   B. health plans
   C. providers
   D. none of the above

3. Which of the following is protected under the HIPAA privacy standards?

   A. patient information communicated over the phone
   B. patient data that is printed and mailed
   C. patient information sent by e-mail
   D. all of the above

4. A Notice of Privacy Practices is given to:

    A. pharmacists
    B. patients
    C. business associates
    D. other covered entities

5. Patients' PHI may be released without authorization to:

    A. family and friends
    B. social workers providing services to the patient
    C. local newspapers
    D. online tabloids

6. Which of the following is an example of fraud?

    A. leaving a field blank on the CMS-1500 by mistake
    B. altering a patient's chart to increase the amount reimbursed
    C. releasing a patient's medical records without the patient's consent to the patient's family because you feel morally obligated to do so
    D. miscoding a diagnosis unintentionally

7. Which of the following medical codes is used to identify drug products?

    A. CPT-4
    B. NDC
    C. HCPCS
    D. CDT-4

8. Which of the following specifies how patient information is protected on computer networks?

    A. HIPAA Privacy Rule
    B. quality control and assurance
    C. Notice of Privacy Practices
    D. Security Rule

9. The Health Insurance Portability and Accountability Act of 1996 deals with the patient's right to:

    A. get information prior to a treatment
    B. refuse treatment
    C. privacy
    D. choose a physician

10. Violations of HIPAA law can result in which of the following penalties?

    A. criminal penalties
    B. civil penalties
    C. both
    D. neither

11. Disclosure of a patient's health information (PHI) usually requires which of the following, except in the case of TPHCO (Treatment, Payment, and Health Care Operations)?

    A. the patient's approval
    B. the physician's approval
    C. the family's approval
    D. all of the above

12. *Protected health information* is defined as the stored information that is identified about:

    A. a federal agency
    B. an insurance provider
    C. a patient
    D. none of the above

13. Title I of HIPAA is referred to as which of the following?

    A. electronic health information transaction standards
    B. privacy and state law preemption
    C. health insurance reform
    D. all of the above

14. Which of the following is referred to as a "covered entity"?

    A. health insurance plans
    B. health-care providers
    C. clearinghouses
    D. all of the above

15. Health-care covered entities include which of the following?

    A. providers
    B. accreditation agencies
    C. lawyers and collection agents
    D. B and C

Fill in the Blank

1. The release of protected health information to any outside entity is referred to as _____.

2. A "Notice of Privacy Practices" explains to patients how their PHI may be _____ and _____ by providers.

3. The Office for Civil Rights enforces civil violations of HIPAA _____ standards.

4. The Employee Retirement Income and Security Act of 1974 (ERISA) regulates _____ -offered health plans.

5. Patients have a right to _____ and the protection of their private health information.

6. Electronic medical records (EMR) are often confused with electronic _____.

7. Criminal penalties, which are usually assessed for intentional misuse of PHI, can be as high as _____ in fines and up to _____ years in prison.

8. The Centers for Medicare and Medicaid Services (CMS) enforce _____ standards.

9. ICD-9-CM codes are used to identify _____ and conditions.

10. Civil penalties for misuse of PHI can be as high as _____ in fines per year if repeated violations occur.

CASE STUDY

A pharmacy technician is asked to fax a patient's PHI to a pharmacy out of state because the patient will be traveling and will need medications there. He confirms the fax number to which he is to send the information. However, when he dials the number on the fax machine, he transposes two of the numbers and the fax goes to a different location than intended.

1. What should the pharmacy technician have included with this fax to ensure that it was received by the correct person?

2. What should the person who received this information do?

RELATED INTERNET SITES

Search for "HIPAA" at these sites for additional information related to this act.

http://aspe.hhs.gov

http://www.aafp.org

http://www.ama-assn.org

http://www.cms.hhs.gov

http://www.hhs.gov

http://www.himssanalytics.org/hc_providers/index.asp

http://www.hipaaadvisory.com

http://www.hipaacompliancejournal.com

http://www.hipaacomply.com

http://www.hipaaps.com

http://www.ocfs.state.ny.us

http://www.privacyrights.org/fs/fs8a-hipaa.htm

REFERENCES

Abood, R. (2005). *Pharmacy Practice and the Law* (4th ed.). Jones and Bartlett.

Fink, J. L., Vivian, J. C., & Bernstein, I. B. (2006). *Pharmacy Law Digest* (40th ed.). Wolters Kluwer Health.

Fred, L. Y. (2005). *Manual for Pharmacy Technicians* (3rd ed.). ASHP.

Hopper, T. (2007). *Mosby's Pharmacy Technicians Principles & Practice* (2nd ed.). Saunders/Elsevier.

Reiss, B. S., & Hall, G. D. (2006). *Guide to Federal Pharmacy Law* (5th ed.). Apothecary Press.

Workplace Safety Laws

OBJECTIVES

Upon completion of this chapter, the reader should be able to:

1. Explain the bloodborne pathogens standard.
2. Summarize the management of post-exposure evaluation and follow-up.
3. Differentiate between disinfection, sanitization, and sterilization procedures.
4. Identify sexual harassment as a form of sexual discrimination.
5. Identify four areas for which standards are mandated by the Occupational Safety and Health Administration (OSHA) for work done in a pharmacy setting.
6. Discuss the role of pharmacists and technicians in following OSHA standards in the pharmacy.
7. Summarize standard precautions.
8. State the purpose of workers' compensation laws.
9. Discuss exposure control plans.
10. Briefly describe the guidelines of an exposure control plan.

KEY TERMS

Airflow hood – A workstation that emits a stream of highly filtered air that reduces possible contamination of the substances being used.

Biohazard symbol – An international symbol that is used to designate any substance harmful to human health, including bloodborne pathogens and medical wastes.

Bloodborne pathogen – Any infectious microorganism present in blood or other body fluids and tissues.

Chemical hygiene plan – A "laboratory standard" established by OSHA to reduce exposures to chemicals when handled by employees.

Compensation claim – A claim filed with the state that addresses an on-site workplace injury or illness.

Federal Register – A U.S. government publication that contains all administrative laws, and is the primary source of information for OSHA standards.

Fire safety plan – A workplace plan detailing locations of fire alarm pull boxes, fire extinguishers, and fire sprinklers, as well as a plan for continued fire prevention training and drills.

Germicides – Agents that kill germs, also known as "disinfectants."

Hazard communication plan – A system of notifying personnel of hazards by applying warning labels that signify the types and ratings of hazardous chemicals and substances.

Hazardous waste – A solid, chemical, radioactive, or infectious material that may transmit pathogens or other hazardous substances.

Material Safety Data Sheet (MSDS) – A form that is required for all hazardous chemicals or other substances that are used in laboratories or pharmacies. This form contains information about a product's name, chemical characteristics, ingredients, guidelines for safe handling, physical and health hazards, and procedures to be followed in the event of exposure.

Medical Waste Tracking Act – An act that gives OSHA the authority to inspect hazardous medical waste and cite offices for unhealthy or unsafe practices regarding them.

Occupational Safety and Health Administration (OSHA) – A division of the U.S. Department of Labor.

Radioactive waste – Any waste that contains or is contaminated with liquid or solid radioactive materials.

Workers' compensation – Laws that establish procedures for compensating workers who are injured on the job, with the employer paying the cost of the insurance premium for the employee.

SETTING THE SCENE

Sheila, a 26-year-old, has been working as a pharmacy technician in a chain pharmacy for 16 months. The pharmacist's name is Brad, and he is Sheila's supervisor. He is 45 years old and was divorced 3 years previously. For some time Brad has been sexually harassing Sheila. Fearing for her job, she doesn't tell anyone after Brad fondles her in the storage room. Upset at what happened, Sheila takes an indefinite sick leave, which leads to Brad firing her.

Critical Thinking

- If you were in Sheila's situation, what would you do?

- After she was fired, what steps do you think Sheila could take?

- Do you think sexual harassment is, in general, considered a felony or a misdemeanor?

OVERVIEW

Many federal and state laws govern the workplace. Federal laws may apply only to those businesses with a certain number of employees (such as 15, 20, or 50) who work for a minimum number of weeks per year. This almost always includes pharmacies. State laws may apply to those areas not covered by federal law, or may extend (or overlap) existing federal law. It is important to note that even small pharmacies that employ fewer than 15 people are usually subject to the Civil Rights Act since they are federal contractors (because they provide services to Medicare or Medicaid).

These laws provide specifically for employee safety and welfare. Major areas include workplace safety regulations, including medical hazard regulations, job-related injuries and illnesses, and unemployment or reemployment. The Occupational Safety and Health Act (OSHA) was developed to maintain a reporting system for job-related injuries and illnesses, and to reduce hazards in the workplace. In the pharmacy, this law affects the following:

- air contaminants
- eye and skin protection
- flammable and combustible liquids
- the hazard communication standard

Safe working conditions must be ensured by pharmacies because biologic, electrical, chemical, and radiation hazards are encountered in pharmacy settings on a daily basis. It is important for pharmacy technicians to be aware of hazards, and to have knowledge about safety precautions. They need to know the rules necessary for eliminating or minimizing hazards.

Occupational Safety and Health Administration (OSHA)

In 1970, President Nixon signed the Occupational Safety and Health Act, which created the Occupational Safety and Health Administration (OSHA). OSHA is a division of the U.S. Department of Labor. Workplace injuries, illnesses, and fatalities have been significantly reduced since OSHA was created. OSHA's mission is to ensure workplace safety and a healthy work environment for all employees.

This act created compulsory standards for health and safety in the workplace, which are enforced by OSHA. It includes regulations for the following:

- Administrative requirements
- First aid
- Machinery and equipment
- Materials
- Physical workplace

- Power sources
- Processing
- Protective clothing

All employees must know the OSHA standards that apply to their business. The Federal Register is a U.S. government publication that contains all administrative laws, and is the primary source of information for OSHA standards.

The Occupational Safety and Health Administration is authorized to do the following:

- Establish "separate but dependent responsibilities and rights" for employers and employees for the achievement of better safety and health conditions
- Encourage employers and employees to reduce workplace hazards and to implement new and improved health programs
- Develop mandatory job safety and health standards, and enforce them effectively
- Maintain a record-keeping system to monitor job-related injuries and illnesses

OSHA established the Occupational Exposure to Hazardous Chemicals Standard and the Bloodborne Pathogens Standard. The primary goal of the Bloodborne Pathogens Standard was to reduce occupational-related cases of HIV and hepatitis B infection among health-care workers.

Occupational Exposure to Hazardous Chemicals Standard

OSHA requires that risk assessments be performed in workplaces that use hazardous chemicals. Standard operating procedures should include the use of protective equipment, clearly defined steps to be taken in case of exposure, storage of antitoxins for emergencies, proper storage of hazardous materials, and approved methods of waste disposal.

The Occupational Exposure to Hazardous Chemicals Standard requires the following tasks to be performed by employers:

1. Inventory any and all hazardous chemicals regarding quantity, manufacturer's name, address, and chemical hazard classification.
2. Assemble MSDS from manufacturers. The sheets should be kept in a manual and regularly reviewed. Label chemicals using the National Fire Protection Association's color and numbering method.

3. Provide educational training to all employees who handle any hazardous materials within 30 days of employment and before an employee is allowed to handle the chemicals.

4. Develop and evaluate a chemical hygiene plan to address how to handle any spills or exposures.

Bloodborne Pathogens Standard

The term **bloodborne pathogen** is applied to any infectious microorganism present in blood or other body fluids and tissues. Bloodborne pathogens are one of the most significant biohazards faced by health-care workers. The most publicized bloodborne pathogens are human immunodeficiency virus (HIV), hepatitis B virus (HBV), and hepatitis C virus (HCV). Though pharmacy technicians usually have less chance of exposure to bloodborne pathogens in the pharmacy setting, they should still have knowledge about the dangers of these pathogens.

OSHA requires medical facilities to comply with the Bloodborne Pathogens Standard, and to prove their compliance to OSHA inspectors if necessary. This standard protects OSHA personnel who may face potential bloodborne pathogen exposure at work, and addresses the following:

1. Control and determination of exposure

2. Universal precautions

3. Hepatitis B virus vaccine in the case of those potentially exposed to bloodborne pathogens while on the job

4. Post-exposure follow-up

5. Labeling and disposal of biologic wastes

6. Housekeeping and laundry functions

7. Employee training

Focus On...

Safety

For the safety of employees and all clients, carefully following and monitoring safety regulations is essential. Job descriptions should identify any position that may cause exposure to hazardous chemicals and bloodborne pathogens.

Aseptic Technique

The goal of aseptic technique is to minimize contamination by pathogens. It involves a carefully controlled, specific set of practices and procedures. Good aseptic technique also protects health-care workers from contamination, as well as patients. Aseptic technique includes the practices of cleaning, sanitizing, and disinfecting to remove impurities on equipment or personnel, and reduce the amount of microorganisms to the greatest possible extent. It is important to use aseptic technique to prevent contamination of an otherwise sterile medication. Aseptic technique is of the utmost importance during surgery, as well as in many other practical applications. Health-care personnel and equipment, as well as the environment, are all capable of transferring microorganisms. In the pharmacy, the use of aseptic technique is generally referred to as "medical asepsis" or "clean technique" for sterile compounding (mainly of parenteral products to decrease risk to patients).

Personal Protective Equipment (PPE)

Under OSHA's guidelines, personal protective equipment (PPE) is used to protect employees from bodily fluids, including blood. It can prevent contamination through the skin, wounds, and mucous membranes. Personal protective equipment includes the following, put on in this sequential order:

- Gowns or lab coats – worn over regular clothing; they may be laundered and reused

- Face shields, goggles, and masks – used when there is a risk of splashing or splattering with bodily fluids; face shields and goggles may be reused; masks may either be single-use or made for multiple uses

- Gloves – used when there is a possibility of hand contamination; gloves are to be used one time only

Eyewash stations should be provided so that workers can wash out their eyes, or flush mucous membranes, with water in cases of accidental exposure to bodily fluids or chemicals. Figure 6-1 shows personal protective equipment, while Figure 6-2 shows an eyewash station.

What Would You Do?

While John was compounding in the laboratory, he was splashed in the eyes with a chemical. He went to the men's room and washed his face in the sink. He did not use the eyewash facilities. After going back to work, he found that his eyes remained irritated, and he could not see very well. If you were John, what would you do in this situation?

Exposure Control Plan

Exposure control plans should be printed so that they can be readily referred to. Per OSHA guidelines, they should be updated

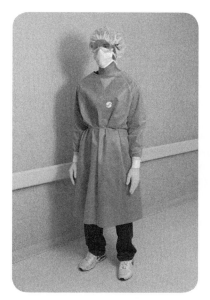

Figure 6-1 Proper personal protective equipment.

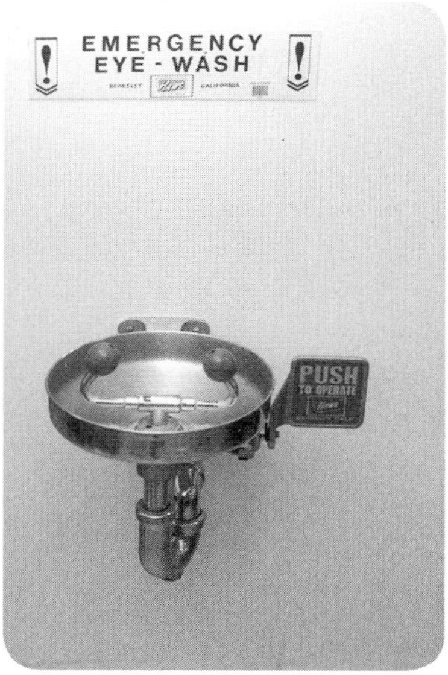

Figure 6-2 Eyewash station.

annually. These plans are intended to lower the risks for exposure to dangerous or infectious materials, and to prevent bloodborne diseases from being transmitted. OSHA has regulations about a variety of hazardous substances, including those that are radioactive. A "universal precautions statement" should be included which explains the type of precautions that are to be taken by every employee who may be exposed to hazards. Exposure control plans usually include the following hazards:

- Sharps
- Bins or pails
- Broken glassware
- Laundry
- Substances used for vaccinations

    Exposure control plans focus on several areas, including:

- The types of exposure that may occur in the workplace
- Personal protective equipment
- Housekeeping requirements for the workplace
- Hepatitis B vaccines at no cost for employees who have had a potential bloodborne pathogen exposure at work

- Warning labeling and training about exposure and post-exposure

- Good documentation concerning medical records, training sessions, and on-the-job injuries

Post-Exposure Procedures

Exposure at the workplace to bloodborne pathogens and other infectious diseases should be discussed in the policies and procedures manual. In general, an exposure incident should be followed up with a medical evaluation of the employee, provided by the employer. Exposure may occur in a variety of ways, including:

- Needle sticks (or sticks from other potentially contaminated sharp objects)

- Splashing of substances into mucous membranes or other body areas

- Contact with intact or non-intact skin

In the pharmacy, exposure can commonly occur during compounding by contact with sharps, splashing, and even inhalation of hazardous substances. Eyewash facilities should be available so that the technician can thoroughly rinse out the body area of possible contamination. Immediately after exposure, clean the area of exposure with water or soap and water (if possible), and inform your supervisor that you need to be evaluated and/or treated because of the exposure.

What Would You Do?

Mary, a pharmacy technician working in a hospital pharmacy, was splashed when she accidentally dropped a glass medication bottle into an airflow hood. The moving air carried the medication onto her face. She was not wearing a mask but was wearing protective glasses. The medication partially entered into her nose. If you were Mary, what would you do in this situation?

Pharmacy Hazard Regulation

Potential hazards in the pharmacy should be addressed by a pharmacy hazard regulation standard. OSHA provides clear instruction about possible hazards as they relate to the practice of pharmacy, and will conduct a free assessment of the workplace upon request. Personnel in the pharmacy should be familiar with OSHA's guidelines concerning hazardous substances, and methods that can help them avoid contamination regardless of the transmission pathway (by inhalation, via the mouth, or through the skin).

Good worker training upon hiring, and thereafter on an annual (or even more regular) schedule, can minimize pharmacy hazards. Specific worker training, focusing on the actual individual job requirements, is critical so that each employee is thoroughly prepared for his or her own job's potential hazards, and with which particular hazardous substances they may come in contact. Re-training may be required if an employee has not received OSHA training for more than 1 year, and is no longer familiar with all of the basic OSHA training requirements related to their workplace. Re-training may be required when an employee changes job duties, because the hazards they must be familiar with may change along with them. When new hazardous substances are introduced into a workplace, it is also recommended that further training be given. After an accident or near-accident occurs, it may also be time for further training.

OSHA generally requires that individuals who teach employees about OSHA safety requirements have the following credentials, related to the individual subjects that they teach:

- Thorough experience with the subject

- Strong knowledge about the subject

- Previous training about the subject prior to their own ability to teach it

In most workplaces, safety managers or supervisors conduct OSHA training. OSHA provides training for instructors through videos and software. The OSHA reference materials library is located at http://www.osha.gov (click on "Compliance Assistance"; "Training and Reference Materials Library").

Along with proper training, the use of warning labels and MSDS also complement a safe pharmacy setting. Chemicals or drugs that are considered hazardous include those that are carcinogenic, corrosive, irritating, sensitizing, or toxic. Every year, an updated list of potentially hazardous drugs is released by the National Institute for Occupational Safety and Health (NIOSH).

You Be the Judge

*A compounding pharmacy provided its workers with gowns, goggles, gloves, and similar equipment on a regular basis, but did not provide an **airflow hood** because the types of substances compounded there did not require such a device. Because of a fire that occurred in a nearby compounding pharmacy, this pharmacy was asked to quickly handle the compounding for cytotoxic agents required for several different patients. A pharmacy technician who knew that an airflow hood was required for these agents refused to complete the compounding, and was reprimanded. He notified OSHA that the pharmacist was completing the compounding of cytotoxic agents without the proper equipment. What do you think the OSHA inspectors would do in this case?*

Chemical Hygiene Plan

OSHA has set forth a "laboratory standard" that was designed to reduce exposures to chemicals by employees. It suggests that a chemical hygiene officer be designated to manage the ways that chemicals are handled in the workplace. A **chemical hygiene plan** should be instituted that details the ways that each employee should handle the chemicals that are used. Included in the plan should be sections that focus on administrative and engineering controls, as well as personal protective equipment. The plan should outline emergency preparedness procedures concerning acceptable and unacceptable procedures, the use of compressed gases, particularly hazardous substances, potential explosions, proper labeling, laminar airflow hoods, and safety equipment.

Fire Safety Plan

Pharmacy technicians and other pharmacy employees should be aware of procedures to follow in case of fire. They should know where fire extinguishers are located, and be familiar with their use. Technicians should also understand how to use fire blankets or heavy toweling to smother fires on clothing. In addition, they should be familiar with the location of emergency exits. Every **fire safety plan** must be compliant with OSHA regulations. These plans should include written (and posted) procedures with clearly marked escape routes. OSHA requires employers to provide the following as part of their fire safety plan:

- Fire alarm pull boxes, tested on a regular basis
- Fire extinguishers
- Fire sprinklers, tested on a regular basis
- Fire prevention training
- Fire drills, conducted on a regular basis

Figure 6-3 shows a clearly marked escape route in the case of a fire.

What Would You Do?

Shannon was working with electronic equipment in her pharmacy when a power cord caught fire. She was extremely nervous, and could not remember what she should do in case of fire. If you were Shannon, what procedures do you think she should follow?

Electrical Safety

Pharmacy technicians must be familiar with electricity and how it relates to the pharmacy setting. All electrical equipment holds the potential for becoming a fire hazard if used improperly or if in poor

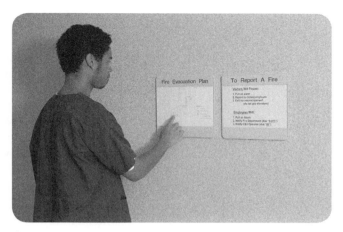

Figure 6-3 Fire evacuation plan.

working condition. Electrical shocks can and do occur, but can be minimized by good training and maintenance of equipment. Extension cords and multi-outlet electrical plugs should be used minimally. Overloaded electrical circuits can result in fires, so outlets should never be overused. Every employee should know the location of the circuit breaker box for the pharmacy. Spills of various drugs or chemicals should be avoided, but especially near electrical outlets, equipment, or power strips.

Radiation Safety

Radioactive waste is any waste that contains or is contaminated with liquid or solid radioactive materials. This waste must be clearly labeled as radioactive and never placed into an incinerator, down a drain, or in public areas. It should be removed only by a licensed removal service.

Radiation hazard symbols are used to inform personnel of areas where radiation is in use. Storage areas of radioactive materials are likewise labeled, as are radioactive material containers. To be safe from radiation, it is important to maintain good standards of radiation exposure protection. Exposure times must be the minimum required for the procedure to be performed. Proper shielding must be worn, and correct distances from the radiation source maintained. Pharmacy technicians must be trained in the use of radioactive materials if they are required to work with them in any manner.

Focus On...

Radiation Safety

Personnel working with radioactive materials must wear a special reactive nametag that measures radiation levels in order to prevent overexposure.

Hazard Communication Plan

A **hazard communication plan** details the hazardous chemicals and substances that are present in the workplace. It explains to employees the potential health risks. Material safety data sheets (MSDS) are part of a hazard communication plan, and pharmacy technicians must be familiar with the MSDS for each chemical or substance used (MSDS will be discussed later in this chapter). Chemicals must be properly contained, sealed, and labeled. Figure 6-4 shows clear and accurate labeling of a chemical in the workplace.

The National Fire Protection Association (NFPA) is the world's primary advocate of fire prevention and safety. Its mission is to set codes and standards, conduct research, and to provide training and education about safety from fire and other hazards. The NFPA provides a colored, numbered hazard identification symbol for every chemical that may be potentially hazardous. The top

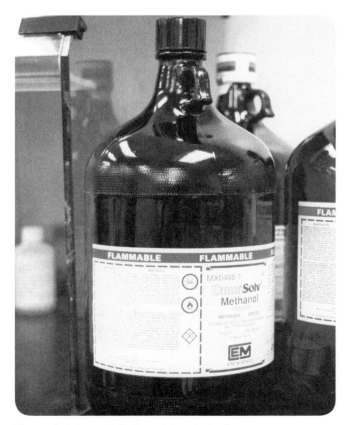

Figure 6-4 Proper labeling of chemical substances.

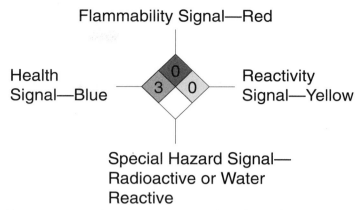

Figure 6-5 National Fire Protection Agency hazard identification symbol.

diamond indicates the flammability potential of the chemical. The left diamond indicates the potential health hazard of the chemical. The right diamond shows the stability or reactivity potential of the chemical. The bottom diamond features specialized information, such as biohazard or radioactivity information. The numbers used in this system range from 0 (meaning "no hazard") to 4 (meaning "extremely hazardous"). The NFPA hazard identification system is demonstrated in Figure 6-5.

Medical Waste Tracking Act

Hospitals, laboratories, pharmacies, nursing homes, and other health-care facilities generate 3.2 million tons of hazardous medical waste each year. Much of this waste is dangerous, especially when it is potentially infectious or radioactive. OSHA may, under the authority of the **Medical Waste Tracking Act**, inspect hazardous medical wastes and cite offices for unhealthy or unsafe practices regarding them.

Hazardous medical wastes include four major types of medical waste: solid, chemical, radioactive, and infectious. An approved sharps container that is puncture-proof must be provided for disposal of sharp objects. These containers are very important for infectious medical wastes such as bloodborne pathogens. Chemical wastes include **germicides**, cleaning solvents, and pharmaceuticals. These wastes can create a hazardous situation (a fire or explosion) in both institutional and community pharmacies. They can also cause harm if ingested, inhaled, or absorbed through the skin or mucous membranes. Pharmacy technicians have a duty to refrain from pouring toxic, flammable, or irritating chemicals down a drain. Chemicals should be discarded only in glass or metal containers. Because of the Resource Conservation and Recovery Act, established by the Environmental Protection Agency (EPA), in most states chemicals cannot be flushed or washed down a drain, even with large quantities of water. Chemical wastes must be documented on an MSDS, which also provides specific information on handling and disposing of chemicals safely.

Other hazardous wastes must be contained in leak-proof, plastic biohazard bags. These materials should be handled by reputable and licensed medical waste handlers. Medical wastes are often disposed of by incineration.

Focus On...

Solid Wastes

Solid waste is not considered hazardous, but can pollute the environment. Mandatory recycling programs have assisted in reducing some of the solid wastes produced in the United States.

Focus On...

The Medical Waste Tracking Act

The federal law that authorizes OSHA to inspect hazardous medical wastes and to cite pharmacies for unsafe or unhealthy practices regarding these wastes is the Medical Waste Tracking Act.

Disposal of Hazardous Materials and Spill Cleanup

Containers that hold hazardous wastes must be labeled with the biohazard symbol to alert employees of the dangers of the materials within. Figure 6-6 shows the biohazard symbol.

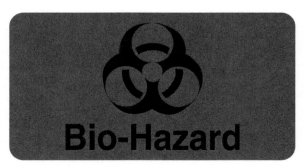

Figure 6-6 Biohazard symbol.

The term "hazardous waste" includes many different substances and materials, including those that have been exposed to blood or body fluids. Other potential hazardous wastes include:

- Gloves and other protective clothing or equipment
- Dressings and equipment from medical procedures
- Paper towels and other cleaning equipment
- Sharps, including needles, syringes, and blades
- Microscope slides

Hazardous waste containers are available in a variety of different sizes and thicknesses, as well as being made from hard or soft plastics and other substances. Pharmacy technicians who work with hazardous waste containers must wear full protective equipment, with general cleaning staff not having access to these containers. Often, an outside company is hired to remove and disposal of all hazardous waste. Laws and regulations concerning the transportation, storage, and handling of hazardous materials can be found at http://phmsa.dot.gov (click on "Hazmat Safety Community"; "Hazardous Materials Information Center").

Figure 6-7 shows hazardous waste containers.

When a spill occurs, the specific policies and procedures of the workplace must be followed carefully. Spill kits are used to properly clean up a variety of spills. These kits contain protective

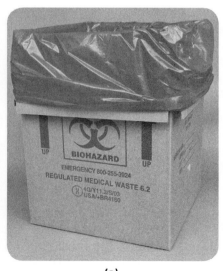

(a)

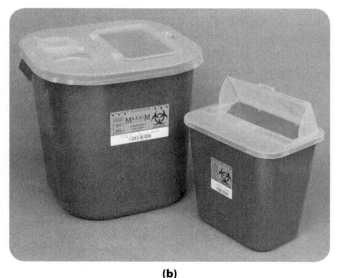

(b)

Figure 6-7 (a) Biohazard and (b) sharps containers.

equipment and clothing that keep workers safe from various types of contamination from materials that may be spilled at work. They usually contain most of the following items:

- Disposable scoops
- Eye protection
- Gauze or toweling (disposable after use)
- Gloves (usually both latex gloves and utility gloves)
- Gowns or coveralls that are disposable after use
- Plastic containers that are leak- and puncture-resistant
- Powder designed for absorption
- Protective equipment
- Respirators
- Sealable bags made of thick plastic
- Shoe covers
- Spill pads
- Warning signs that a spill has occurred

When a spill occurs, all broken fragments from containers and equipment should be put into thick plastic bags or containers. Liquid substances should be absorbed using pads or towels. Dry substances such as powders should be cleaned up with wet gauze or towels. The spill area should be rinsed off with water. Then, a detergent should be used to wash the area, followed by a second rinse with water. Work from the outer edges of the spill, moving inward. If the area is carpeted, special absorbent powder is often used to lift the spilled substances from the carpeting. It is important to have special vacuum cleaners on hand that are to be used only for hazardous materials that have been spilled. Every spill should be documented in an incident report and filed at the workplace. OSHA forms that are used for reporting and summarizing work-related injuries and illnesses can be found at http://www.osha.gov (click on "Recordkeeping").

Training and Accident Report Documentation

Each pharmacy must have a written training program detailing how pharmacy technicians will be provided with information and training related to workplace hazards. OSHA dictates that training should include information about hazards in the work area, locations of hazard lists and MSDS manuals, and explanations of MSDS manuals and hazardous chemical labeling systems, as well as any measures that pharmacy technicians may use to protect themselves. Training logs should be kept, signed, and dated upon completion of each type of training. Accident reports are required if accidents occur and must contain:

- The pharmacy's name and address
- The pharmacy technician's name, address, and phone number
- Where, when, and how the accident occurred, and what was involved
- The nature of the injury
- Medical treatment, hospitalization, or other follow-up information

A log of all occupational injuries and illness must be kept for 5 years following the end of the calendar year to which they relate by employers, and these must be available for inspection by the U.S. Department of Health and Human Services, the U.S. Department of Labor, and state officials. OSHA health-care setting standards may be obtained from state or regional OSHA offices, or from OSHA at:

U.S. Department of Labor, Occupational Safety and Health Administration
Directorate of Health Standards Programs
200 Constitution Avenue NW
Washington, D.C. 20210.

What Would You Do?

Mark is a pharmacy technician. Three weeks after he was hired, his pharmacist set up an OSHA training class. Mark was sick during this time, and unable to attend. On his first day back at work, he was attempting to clean up a corrosive chemical spill on the floor. Since he had missed the training, Mark was unsure of the proper procedures to follow, and wore latex gloves while cleaning up the spill. If you were Mark, what would you do in this situation?

OSHA Record Keeping Regulation

OSHA may make unannounced visits to the workplace, and may issue citations or penalties of up to $1,000 per violation to an employer who does not provide a safe environment. The OSHA regulations contain a clinical hygiene plan that addresses training, information requirements, and provisions that must be implemented for chemical exposure in the pharmacy setting. Chemical inventories must be taken, and material safety data sheets (MSDS) are to be provided by sellers of particular products to purchasers.

An MSDS is a form that is required for all hazardous chemicals or other substances that are used in laboratories or pharmacies. This form contains information about a product's name, chemical characteristics, ingredients, guidelines for safe handling, physical and health hazards, and procedures to be followed in the event of exposure. An MSDS manual should be assembled by the employer that contains all of the material safety data sheets pertinent to the workplace.

Employers are required to provide a hazard communication program to employees within 30 days of hire. A hazard communication program is designed to inform employees about hazardous substances in the workplace, their potential harmful effects, and appropriate control measures.

Violations of OSHA

The most common violations of Occupational Safety and Health Administration regulations include the following:

- No eyewash facilities available at facilities that are required to have them
- No labeling (or improper labeling) of hazardous chemicals
- No MSDS for each hazardous chemical

Employee Responsibilities

Some states follow OSHA regulations regarding the responsibilities of employees, while others adopt their own regulations. Employees are not directly cited by OSHA when they breach the organization's regulations. However, in most states, regulations are similar to those established by OSHA concerning employee responsibilities. Employees should familiarize themselves with the following so that they understand their responsibilities:

- They should read all OSHA posters
- They should follow all OSHA standards for proper compliance
- They should follow the regulations of their employer concerning the use of protective equipment while at work
- They should report any hazardous conditions to their supervisor
- They should report any on-the-job injuries or illnesses to their supervisor and ask for prompt treatment
- They should cooperate with any OSHA inspectors if they are questioned about the workplace safety and health conditions
- They should understand and exercise their rights as set forth by OSHA

You Be the Judge

Joshua took a special OSHA course and understood his responsibilities on the job. One day, he was doing his routine work and dealing with chemical substances. He did not use protective equipment for safety. What could be the result of Joshua's actions?

WORKERS' COMPENSATION

Workers' compensation laws establish procedures for compensating workers who are injured on the job, with the employer paying the cost of the insurance premium for the employee. These state and federal laws allow claims for compensation to be filed with state or federal governments instead of suing. The laws require workers to accept workers' compensation as the exclusive remedy for on-the-job injuries. Federal laws cover workers in Washington, D.C., coal miners, federal employees, and maritime workers. State laws cover those workers not protected under federal statutes. There are five types of state compensation benefits for which workers may apply:

1. Medical (hospital, medical and surgical services, medications, and prosthetic devices) treatment

2. Temporary disability indemnity (weekly cash payments to the injured or ill employee)

3. Permanent disability indemnity (either a lump sum award or a weekly or monthly cash payment)

4. Death benefits for survivors (consisting of cash payments to dependants of employees killed while on-the-job)

5. Rehabilitation benefits (which are paid for vocational or medical rehabilitation)

One area of concern in the pharmacy workplace is in the physical design of the facility, and how it relates to the employees' ability to conduct normal day-to-day tasks without straining their backs, legs, arms, etc. This includes an ergonomic design so that items may be easily reached and are not too high to be easily accessed by the employees. Packages should not be of excessive size or weight so that strains are not caused by lifting or moving them. Easy-access shelving, work areas, and comfortable seating all combine to contribute to a healthy, ergonomic work environment that helps to avoid needless employee injury.

The individual states have different regulations concerning workers' compensation cases for pharmacy employees. Make sure you know your pharmacy policy in accordance with the rules of your state. Records management of workers' compensation varies by state. Injuries or illnesses because of the workplace must be reported immediately to a worker's supervisor. An injury report and compensation claim are then filed with the correct state workers' compensation agency, as well as forms from the attending or designated physician who examines and treats the employee. A pharmacy employee may be required to file the physician's report with the state workers' compensation agency. Each state has different requirement concerning waiting periods and other filing specifics. When a claim is filed, all questions must be fully and thoroughly answered.

Workers' compensation originated shortly after the turn of the 20th century, and was amongst the first social insurance programs. Most states had adopted workers' compensation laws by 1920. Before these laws, workers who were injured on the job could ask their employers for compensation for their injuries, but there was no guaranteed outcome to their requests. Many employers avoided paying for their workers' injuries by claiming that the workers understood job-related dangers and hazards, and accepted these working conditions when they were employed. Some workers accepted more dangerous jobs for higher pay, resulting in no compensation from their employers when an accident occurred.

After workers' compensation laws were enacted, most claims no longer required the worker to prove that the employer was at fault and therefore responsible for the injuries they sustained. After an injury, most employees could receive up to two-thirds of their weekly pay while they were recovering. Families of workers who died on the job would usually receive reimbursement for burial costs, plus up to two-thirds of the deceased worker's weekly pay, every week, up to a pre-determined total amount.

Focus On...

Workers' Compensation

Workers' compensation is a form of insurance established by federal and state statutes that provides reimbursement for workers who are injured on-the-job.

SEXUAL HARASSMENT

Sexual harassment occurs in a variety of circumstances. Anyone may be sexually harassed. A man or a woman may be either the victim or the harasser. A victim and their harasser do not need to be of the opposite sex. A victim may be either the person actually being harassed or even a co-worker who overhears the harassment.

The Civil Rights Act of 1964 protects employees from sexual harassment that occurs on the job. The employer is strictly liable for the acts of supervisors who sexually harass employees that they are in charge of, as well as for some acts of harassment by co-workers and clients. Employers must provide a written policy on sexual harassment.

Written pharmacy policies about sexual harassment should include the following:

1. A statement that sexual harassment of employees will not be tolerated

2. A statement that any employee who feels harassed must bring the matter to the immediate attention of specially designated person within the company

3. A statement about the confidentiality of all related incidents and specific disciplinary action against harassers

4. Procedures that will be followed if harassment occurs

Traditionally, sexual harassment has involved the trading of sexual favors for advancement or rewards within a company. Sexual harassment is a form of discrimination. It is the responsibility of all employees not to discriminate against their fellow employees in any manner, including sexual harassment. Sexual questions, comments, jokes, or inappropriate touching also fall under the heading of sexual harassment. An employer who does not correct these forms of sexual harassing behavior is liable under Title VII of the Civil Rights Act. The Equal Employment Opportunity Act of 1972 gave the Equal Employment Opportunity Commission (EEOC) the power to enforce Title VII. In 1977, the Washington, D.C. Circuit Court ruled that "quid pro quo" (something given for something received) sexual harassment is sexual discrimination.

The steps in stopping sexual harassment are suggested in the following order:

1. Tell the harasser to stop the behavior.

2. Tell another colleague or threaten the harasser that you will tell another person – your Human Resources representatives are usually the best initial choice, followed by senior management. Your employee handbook should list the steps that you can take.

3. Document the harassment.

4. If no help is given from your company, seek legal advice.

Individuals who are prosecuted for sexual harassment can receive a variety of consequences if their actions are proven. These include loss of employment (which may seriously affect future employment opportunities), fines, imprisonment, remedial classes, court costs, and publication throughout the community of the individual's actions. Web sites exist today that publish the names, photos, and addresses of convicted sexual offenders of many different types. An example of this type of Web site is http://www.familywatchdog.us.

What Would You Do?

Richard was talking to one of his co-workers, Nicole, in the pharmacy. He told her a rather rude joke of a sexual nature. Nicole was offended by the joke. If you were Nicole, what would you do?

SUMMARY

Federal and state laws specifically provide for employee safety and welfare. These laws include workplace safety regulations. Congress passed the Occupational Safety and Health Act in 1970 to prevent workplace disease and injuries. This act includes regulations for the physical workplace, machinery and equipment, materials, power sources, processing, protective clothing, first aid, and administrative requirement.

In the pharmacy, personal protective equipment should be used by pharmacy technicians. They should be familiar with their pharmacy's exposure control plan, and follow post-exposure procedures. Safety in the pharmacy should be maintained by establishing and following fire, electrical, and radiation safety plans. OSHA has established record-keeping methods that must be followed concerning exposure to hazardous materials, as well as fire and safety training documentation.

OSHA may make unannounced visits to the workplace and may issue citations or penalties of up to $1,000 per violation to employers who do not provide safe environments. OSHA may also, under the authority of the Medical Waste Tracking Act, inspect hazardous medical wastes and cite pharmacies or medical offices for unhealthy or unsafe practices regarding them.

Each employer must have a written training program detailing how employees will be provided with information about hazards in the work area, locations of hazard lists and MSDS manuals, and hazardous chemical labeling systems. Hazardous materials must be disposed of properly, by using protective equipment, approved containers, and correct labeling. Special removal agencies are usually used to transfer hazardous materials out of the workplace. Common hazardous chemicals found in the pharmacy include: pharmaceuticals such as epinephrine, nitroglycerin, physostigmine salicylate, chemotherapy agents, reserpine, chromium, and more.

Pharmacy technicians should have information about workers' compensation in case any on-the-job injuries occur. They should understand the correct methods of filing workers compensation claims and understand the benefits of their pharmacy's plan. The Civil Rights Act protects employees from sexual harassment that occurs on the job. Employers must provide a written policy on this matter.

SETTING THE SCENE

The following discussion and responses relate to the opening "Setting the Scene" scenario:

- Sheila should have told Brad to stop all of the harassment or she would report him to the proper authorities.

- Sheila could file a sexual harassment lawsuit against Brad.

- Sexual harassment is, in most jurisdictions, considered a serious misdemeanor unless it involves physical violence or rape, in which case it is a felony.

REVIEW QUESTIONS

Multiple Choice

1. How long must pharmacies keep logs of occupational injuries available for inspection?

   A. 1 year
   B. 3 years
   C. 5 years
   D. 10 years

2. Workers' compensation includes which of the following types of laws?

   A. state law
   B. federal law
   C. both state and federal law
   D. civil (private) law

3. Which legislation protects against sexual harassment?

    A. OSHA
    B. Equal Employment Opportunity Act
    C. Civil Rights Act
    D. both B and C

4. The blue quadrant of the National Fire Protection Association diamond-shaped symbol for hazardous materials indicates:

    A. health hazard
    B. fire hazard
    C. reactivity hazard
    D. specific hazard

5. The OSHA regulations contain a clinical hygiene plan that addresses which of the following?

    A. training and provisions that must be implemented for chemical exposure in the pharmacy setting
    B. training and information requirements that must be implemented for equipment and computer parts
    C. training and information requirements that must be provided for pharmacy technicians to be licensed
    D. all of the above

6. Which of the following is required for accident reports when accidents occur?

    A. pharmacy's name and address
    B. when, where, and how the accident occurred
    C. the nature of the injury
    D. all of the above

7. OSHA may issue citations or penalties of up to _____ per violation to employers who do not provide safe environments.

    A. $1,000
    B. $5,000
    C. $10,000
    D. $50,000

8. The general purpose of OSHA 1970 is to require all employers to ensure employee:

    A. security and a clean environment
    B. safety and health
    C. enjoyment and productivity
    D. none of the above

9. Radioactive wastes should be removed by which of the following methods?

    A. placing them into an incinerator
    B. pouring them down the drain
    C. storing them in public areas
    D. a licensed removal service

10. All of the following are state compensation benefits that may be applied for, except:

    A. medical treatment
    B. rehabilitation benefits
    C. death benefits for survivors
    D. exemptions from state and federal taxes

11. Standard precautions should be followed if the pharmacy technician is exposed to which of the following?

    A. chemical materials
    B. human body fluids
    C. dangerous gases
    D. radioactive substances

12. When pharmacy technicians change hazardous waste bags, they must wear:

    A. protective collars
    B. protective shoes
    C. gowns
    D. gloves

13. OSHA requires that employers with greater than 10 employees:

    A. must record injuries that happen to their employees at home
    B. maintain records of all work-related injuries and illnesses
    C. keep records only if they feel it necessary
    D. maintain vacation records

14. Pharmacies must provide safety training to pharmacy technicians:

    A. upon firing them
    B. upon hiring them
    C. at least once a month
    D. if they are expectant mothers

15. Which of the following forms is required for all hazardous chemicals or substances used in the pharmacy?

A. CMS-1500
B. IRS Form 941
C. TRICARE
D. MSDS

Fill in the Blank

1. OSHA was developed to maintain a reporting system for job-related _____ and reduce hazards in the _____.

2. Hazardous medical wastes include four major types of medical waste: solid, chemical, infectious, and _____.

3. Radioactive waste must be clearly _____ as radioactive and never placed into an incinerator, down a drain, or in _____ areas.

4. Record management of workers' compensation varies by _____.

5. Eyewash stations should be available for _____ decontamination if a technician is exposed to _____ or blood substances.

6. Biohazard symbols alert the pharmacy technician to _____ materials.

7. Proper personal protective _____ must be worn at all times.

8. The single most important means of preventing the spread of infection is _____ and _____ hand hygiene by all pharmacy technicians.

9. Each MSDS contains basic information about the specific _____ or product.

10. The exposure control plan is designed to minimize risk of exposure to _____ material and bloodborne disease.

CASE STUDY

Brian is a pharmacy technician who was asked by his supervisor to take compounded medicinal fluids to a local nursing home.

On the way, he was involved in a car accident that was not his fault and injured. He was hospitalized for 1 week with mild head injuries and a fractured left leg. After being released from the hospital, he had to do physical therapy for 4 months. Though he lost a total of 4½ months from work, Brian did not have any health insurance.

1. Who must Brian report to in order to obtain workers' compensation?

2. Who must pay for Brian's medical expenses?

3. What must Brian's supervisor do on his behalf?

RELATED INTERNET SITES

http://phmsa.dot.gov; click on "Hazmat Safety Community"; "Hazardous Materials Information Center"

http://www.cdc.gov

http://www.eeoc.gov

http://www.epa.gov

http://www.familywatchdog.us

http://www.lbl.gov

http://www.osha.gov

http://www.osha.gov; click on "Recordkeeping"

http://www.oshatrain.org

http://www.workerscompensation.com

REFERENCES

Fink, J. L., Vivian, J. C., & Bernstein, I. B. (2006). *Pharmacy Law Digest* (40th ed.). Wolters Kluwer Health.

Moini, J. (2005). *The Pharmacy Technician – A Comprehensive Approach*. Thomson/Delmar Learning.

STATE LAWS AFFECTING PHARMACY PRACTICE

State Laws and Pharmacy Practice

OUTLINE

OBJECTIVES

Upon completion of this chapter, the reader should be able to:

1. Briefly describe the processing of prescriptions.

2. Explain the role of pharmacy technicians in the processing of prescriptions.

3. List drug labeling requirements.

4. Explain state law as it relates to pharmacy ownership.

5. Discuss patient records and drug review.

6. List computer regulations.

7. Give the minimum requirements for a pharmacy.

8. Define electronic files.

9. Describe patient counseling under OBRA-90.

10. Explain prescription drug orders.

KEY TERMS

Auxiliary labels – Labels applied to drug containers that supply additional information, such as whether to take the medication with or without food, potential adverse effects, to avoid taking with alcohol, etc.

DEA number – A series of numbers assigned to a health-care practitioner that allows him or her to write prescriptions for controlled substances.

Down time – A period of time when a computer or computer system is not operational, for any of a variety of reasons.

Drug history – A history of a patient's medication use over a reasonable period of time, usually for at least the last 5 years; it includes all documented information on prescription medications, non-prescription (OTC) medications, and supplements.

Fax paper – A special paper that burns a thermal image of a transmitted document without using regular paper and printer ink or toner; this type of paper usually causes the burned text and/or images to fade over time.

NDC number – A product identifier used for drugs intended for human use; "NDC" stands for "National Drug Code".

Pharmacy compounding – Creating a new mixture or compound by blending or mixing two or more medications and other substances in a licensed pharmacy.

SETTING THE SCENE

Mrs. Johnstone brings a prescription to your pharmacy. As a pharmacy technician, you realize that she is covered by Medicaid. You dispense her prescription, the pharmacist checks it, and she initials the prescription. Mrs. Johnstone takes her medication and leaves the pharmacy.

Critical Thinking

- What should the pharmacist have done differently to best benefit the patient?

- Did she ignore any state or federal laws? Explain fully.

- If the patient had a severe adverse effect and ended up in the emergency department, who would be responsible: the pharmacist, physician, pharmacy technician, or patient?

OVERVIEW

State laws vary widely. They regulate pharmacy practice, minimum requirements, and how pharmacists and pharmacy technicians are qualified so that they can legally practice. Pharmacists and pharmacy technicians must learn and understand how their state laws differ from federal law, which is regularly addressed in most publications of the industry. Under state laws, pharmacists must be licensed, and must follow the rules and regulations of their state board of pharmacy. In each state, this agency determines how prescriptions are processed, how practitioners may place drug orders, and how the DEA will handle the use of controlled substances. The use of computerized dispensing systems is now the standard in many practices because of improved dispensing time, accuracy, and crosschecking of information.

Most states have their own unique regulations for electronic transmission of prescriptions, usually requiring the prescriber's full information to appear. Drug product selection laws, drug product substitution laws, or generic substitution laws are designed to regulate how pharmacists may dispense a different drug product than the one that was prescribed. Both state and federal laws have enacted "mandatory" Medicaid patient counseling requirements by pharmacists. OBRA-90 dictates how pharmacists must counsel Medicaid patients, be it in person or by telephone. The practice of pharmacy compounding is also regulated by OBRA-90, which limits payments for unlabeled indications. This may affect compounded prescriptions under Medicaid but, otherwise, there is no actual restriction on the practice of compounding.

Pharmacists and pharmacy technicians must understand both their state and federal laws that regulate the practice of pharmacy. They must monitor prescriptions to make sure that prescribers are writing prescriptions within their scope of practice. Confidentiality is of the utmost importance in protecting the protected health information (PHI) of all patients. It is the pharmacist's responsibility to review patient records to determine that there is no misuse of medications.

STATE LAWS AFFECTING PHARMACY PRACTICE

Pharmacists and pharmacy technicians need to be informed about the state and federal regulations that regulate pharmacy practice. The FDA regulates medications, including controlled substances, and medical devices. State agencies, including the state boards of pharmacy, regulate pharmacy practice on a daily basis.

State laws vary widely, however. Because of this, the *National Association of Boards of Pharmacy (NABP)* has created informative, well-organized tables of information that enable pharmacists and pharmacy technicians to quickly find their state's position on a variety of pharmacy-related activities. These tables include information about boards of pharmacy, examination requirements, internships, registration, training, licensure, transfers, renewals, continuing education, disciplinary actions, status of pharmacy technicians, places of practice, wholesaling, distributing, drug control, drug product selection, prescription requirements, transmissions, patient counseling, prescribers, non-controlled and controlled substances, and more.

The NABP developed and published the *Model Pharmacy Practice Act* to promote, preserve, and protect the public safety, health, and welfare by effectively controlling and regulating the practice of pharmacy. This act addresses the licensure of pharmacists, registration of pharmacy technicians, and control of the activities of all people or businesses that manufacture, sell, or distribute drugs or devices used in the dispensing of drugs, along with many other equipment and materials related to the pharmacy field.

What Would You Do?

Tara is a pharmacy technician who recently moved from Maine to Florida. According to the National Association of Boards of Pharmacy, if you were Tara, what must you do in order to be able to practice in Florida? (For reference, see Chapter 8.)

Minimum Requirements for a Pharmacy

Pharmacies are required to have enough space to conduct all of their needed activities, and must have designated patient counseling areas. These are not required to be separate rooms, but simply areas where patient counseling may occur without too much distraction or interference from normal pharmacy activities. They must supply reference materials for patients that educate them about medications and other products. Drug storage must be controlled and orderly, with proper temperature and storage requirements.

All facilities, equipment, and personnel must adhere to OSHA requirements. Proper sinks must be installed, with hot and cold running water. A comprehensive security system must be in place. A complete fire-safety plan, with training of all pharmacy staff, must be in place. A hazard communication plan must be established. The pharmacy must be completely stocked with needed equipment and supplies.

Patients must be able to privately disclose their protected health information. There must always be a pharmacist on duty when the pharmacy is open, though a sign may be placed at the counter for short periods if the pharmacist is temporarily unavailable. Quality control and training programs must be in place. Policies and procedures manuals must be created and followed in an orderly fashion. Licensure must be maintained continually. Prescription drug orders must be received, verified, and processed in a manner consistent with the rules of pharmacy practice set forth by the state board of pharmacy. Equivalent drug products (those that are therapeutically equivalent) may be substituted unless "no substitution allowed" is included on the prescriber's prescription.

All drug products must be properly labeled so that they conform to state board of pharmacy requirements. A thorough patient record system must be in place. Prospective drug use reviews must be conducted as needed. A system of disposal of hazardous materials and biohazards must be in place. Unprofessional conduct must be reported to the proper authorities, as directed by the state board of pharmacy.

You Be the Judge

A new drug store was about to open in Minnesota. The pharmacist tried to follow the minimum requirements of his state. The store opened and, soon after, was inspected by the State Board of Pharmacy. The inspector discovered that the fire safety and hazard communication plans were not in place. What would be the consequences of this situation?

PROCESSING OF PRESCRIPTIONS

The role of pharmacy technicians in the processing of prescriptions requires concentration in order to ensure that all steps are completed properly. According to state law, when a prescription is submitted to a pharmacy for processing, the pharmacy technician must do the following:

- Receive the prescription and verify that all of the information it contains is completed and clear so that it will be correctly filled; prescriptions may be written on prescription pads in handwriting, sent electronically to the pharmacy, or even called in by telephone; in some states, only licensed pharmacists or pharmacist interns can take in prescriptions over the phone

- Translate the prescription so that the information it indicates can be correctly entered into the computer system, and so that the prescription can be labeled with clear instructions for the patient; if there is any question about what was intended by the prescriber, he or she should be called and asked for clarification

- Enter the prescription information into the computer system correctly and completely; make sure that the information in the computer matches the printed labels (one for the medication container and one for the packaging that holds the container) exactly – the pharmacist should initial both of these labels, either via computer or by hand, after verifying that they are correct

- Verify the patient's insurance information and eligibility; if the patient has Medicaid, the prescription must be written on a tamper-proof prescription blank, with some states requiring special prescription blanks for controlled substances

- Fill the prescription and verify that it is correct and packaged according to the standards of the pharmacy and state law; the label should be sent to the counter for filling only after it has been checked with the original order

- Pharmacy technicians should check the stock bottle's labeling and the National Drug Code (**NDC number**) in the computer system, and compare them to the original prescription – it is good practice that stock bottles should be marked with an "X" across the front label, which lets other employees know that the bottle has already been opened and no longer contains the entire labeled amount

    - Never touch the medication when dispensing it
    - Verify that the correct type of lid is affixed onto the correct container properly and firmly

- Check the labels against the original order and, if correct, apply one to the medication container, and one to the packaging that holds the container (usually a bag that is made of paper) – make sure labels are completely intact, not smeared, and placed evenly
- Apply auxiliary labels that may be required by specific medications – these labels, chosen by the pharmacist, may include instructions about certain adverse effects, if the medication should be taken with or without food, and interactions; Figure 7-1 shows examples of auxiliary labels
- Verify that the packaging is correct and initial it
- Put the packaged medication on the original prescription so that the pharmacist can verify them both – in total, the prescription should be checked and verified at least three times during the filling process

The pharmacist can then counsel the patient about the prescription and make sure that he or she understands everything about the proper administration of the drug contained within. The pharmacist is the only person allowed to conduct patient counseling, and pharmacy technicians must always refer patients to the pharmacist whenever they have a question about a prescription.

Computerized dispensing systems can greatly improve dispensing time and accuracy, because they contain many built-in functions that crosscheck and verify information. They also interact with computer inventories to give an up-to-the-minute accounting of all medications in stock. These systems can interact with robotic dispensing equipment to instruct the machinery which medications, amounts, strengths, and forms need to be dispensed.

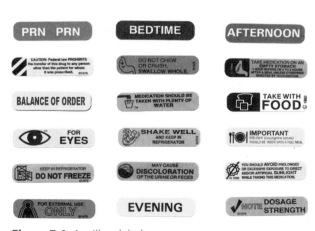

Figure 7-1 Auxiliary labels.

Focus On...

Schedule II Prescriptions

Faxed prescriptions for Schedule II drugs must be followed up by a written prescription; these written follow-ups must be received by the pharmacy within 7 days after the faxed Schedule II prescription was submitted. Faxed prescriptions are allowed for nursing homes or hospice without a written follow-up in some states.

What Would You Do?

Tina, a pharmacy technician, was dispensing a sulfa drug prescription. She forgot to put a required auxiliary label onto the container. The pharmacist noticed that there was no auxiliary label and told Tina that she must put the appropriate label onto the container. If you were Tina, what should you know about sulfa drugs and related auxiliary labels?

Prescription Drug Orders

State law regulates prescribers of medications. Each practitioner, be they a physician, osteopath, dentist, or podiatrist, must be state-licensed. If required, they must also register with the Drug Enforcement Agency (DEA) – all individuals who prescribe controlled substances, for example, must be registered with the DEA. In some states, certified nurse practitioners, physician's assistants, and even pharmacists may prescribe medications. Certain states allow these individuals to prescribe all forms of legal drugs, while others allow them to prescribe all non-controlled substances.

Prescription drug orders should be written by prescribers for diseases and conditions with which they directly deal – for example, a dentist should not be prescribing medication for back pain. Pharmacists should be aware of any prescription that appears to be outside the scope of practice of the prescriber. The amount of a controlled substance should be within the standards of accepted prescribed amounts for a given condition. Doses and combinations of drugs should be looked at closely. Patients who seem to ask for refills more frequently than is normally accepted should be questioned, and their refills investigated if they seem out of the ordinary.

Prescription drug orders for controlled substances should contain the standard information of all other prescriptions, with the addition of the prescriber's DEA number. They should only bear the date of issue, and not any previous dates or post-dates. The practitioner who wrote the prescription must sign the prescription on the actual date of issue, by hand, and not use a stamp that bears the likeness of his or her signature.

Electronic Files

Most states have adopted their own regulations for the electronic transmission of prescriptions. Most states now allow controlled substance prescriptions to be faxed, though individual states have their own restrictions such as requiring that the prescription is written in the prescriber's own handwriting, the inclusion of the actual pharmacy's name that will be filling the order, or that the prescription can only be written for patients in certain health-care settings.

Most states require the prescriber's full information to appear. Prescriptions that are faxed and received on machines using **fax paper** (and not plain paper) must be immediately photocopied onto regular computer printer paper to prevent the fax paper from fading before it can be used. The regulation of computer transmission of prescriptions is changing regularly, as the use of these transmissions of prescriptions becomes more popular.

Drug Product Selection

Drug product selection laws, drug product substitution laws, or generic substitution laws are designed to regulate the ability of pharmacists to dispense a different drug product than the drug that was prescribed. A good amount of cost savings can be attained by the substitution of generic drugs for brand name drugs. The law requires that the generic drug must be identical to the generic drug contained in the brand name drug in order for the substitution to be allowed. If a generic drug is prescribed, the pharmacist can dispense any product that is pursuant to a generically written prescription.

Labeling

Though differences exist in drug labeling requirements between hospital settings, institutional settings, and others, these requirements are, in general, as follows:

- Single-unit packages of individual-dose or unit-dose drug products must include:
    - The drug's generic or trade name
    - The route of administration if other than oral
    - The strength and volume of the drug (preferably in metric measurements)
    - The drug's control number and expiration date
    - The re-packager's name or license number (which must be clearly distinguishable from the rest of the label information)
    - Any special storage conditions
- Multiple-use drug packages must include:
    - Identifying information about the dispensing pharmacy
    - The patient's name
    - The dispensing date
    - The generic and/or trade name of the drug
    - The strength of the drug (preferably in metric measurements)
- Ambulatory or outpatient drug packages must include:
    - The name and address of the dispensing pharmacy
    - The name of the patient
    - The name of the prescriber
    - Directions for use
    - The dispensing date
    - Any federal or state cautions
    - The prescription number
    - The name or initials of the dispensing pharmacist
    - The generic or trade name of the drug
    - The strength of the drug (if more than one strength of the drug is available)
    - The manufacturer or distributor of the drug
    - The beyond-use date of the drug

Focus On...

Labels for Stock Medications

The manufacturer's label found on stock medication bottles contains information about the size of the bottle, the strength of the medication, expiration date, NDC number, and other important facts necessary for providing the correct and safe medication needed by the patient.

Patient Records and Drug Review

The maintenance of patient medication records is intended to facilitate the monitoring of the patient's drug therapy. Good record keeping is important. These records can indicate that the patient was properly counseled by the pharmacist, and that the pharmacist may have contacted the prescriber about possible problems concerning the patient's prescription or prescriptions.

Patient records should contain his or her full name, address, and telephone number. The patient's age or birthdate should be included, as well as gender. Each pharmacy should make sure that every patient record shows his or her entire available **drug history**, of at least the past 5 years, with most recent prescriptions listed first. Any comments by pharmacists should be included, including information about any allergies, reactions, diseases, and conditions.

Focus On...

Protected Health Information

Protected health information should be released from the patient's history only upon the approval of the patient or his or her authorized representative.

The pharmacist has the responsibility to review each patient's medication use and verify that there is no abuse or misuse of medications. The patient's allergies must always be verified to avoid medication errors, and potential interactions with other medications, foods, or supplements avoided. Certain medications are not indicated for certain diseases or conditions, and these must be carefully evaluated. Drug dosages must be checked for effectiveness, and the duration that the medication should be taken must be appropriate. Overuse or underuse of medications should be prevented, and there should be no unneeded duplication of medications. All of these verifications lead to quality therapeutic care and prevent harm to the patient.

Patient Counseling

Patient counseling is to be performed only by licensed pharmacists – not pharmacy technicians or any other pharmacy staff members. Under OBRA-90, most states have enacted "mandatory" patient counseling requirements for pharmacists. These requirements are expanding the pharmacist's standards of practice. OBRA-90 requires pharmacists to offer counseling to all Medicaid patients. It is wise for pharmacists to provide patient counseling in order to ensure that each patient understands the possible adverse effects, drug and food interactions, contraindications, and warnings concerning each prescription. During patient counseling, the pharmacist must explain the name of the drug, its dosage form, its route of administration, the duration of the drug therapy, directions for use, and side effects. The pharmacist should also emphasize how to properly store the medication, and discuss refill information should a refill be required.

Focus On...

Patient Counseling

Pharmacists are required to offer counseling to all Medicaid patients in person, by telephone, or in writing, about his or her prescription medications (according to the individual laws of each state).

COMPUTER REGULATIONS

Secure computer systems are required more than ever for pharmacy record keeping. The National Association of Boards of Pharmacy (NABP) publishes rules for the use of computer systems for the protection and confidentiality of protected health information. PHI must be able to be retrieved online for all prescriptions that may be refilled. All prescription and refill information must be able to be printed out, and include the complete medication history of a given patient. Computer systems of pharmacy record keeping must have secure backup systems in place should the primary system become compromised or unable to be accessed. Pharmacists have final authority and responsibility to make sure that the correct decisions are made for patient refills if an automated computer system is not in proper operation, and any prescriptions filled or refilled during computer "down time" must be entered into the system when it becomes operable within four business days.

PHARMACY OWNERSHIP

Though state laws may restrict who is allowed to own a pharmacy, these restrictions are rare. In general, anyone who has proven their qualifications and is of good moral character may own a pharmacy in most states. The ownership of a pharmacy is usually only of concern if any of the following conditions exists:

- Unlicensed or untrained individuals manage the pharmacy
- A physician owns a pharmacy that causes a conflict of interest with his or her medical practice

- Unethical or undignified pharmacy practices are conducted
- Incorrect or uninformed drug stocking practices are conducted

SALE OF HYPODERMIC NEEDLES AND SYRINGES

The sale of hypodermic needles and syringes must be carefully controlled by the pharmacist to avoid them being used illegally. Individual states regulate the sale of OTC needles and syringes, with some requiring that they be sold only if prescribed by a physician. Other states allow that needles and syringes can be legally purchased without a prescription as long as the patient is at least 18 years of age. These states require that pharmacies not advertise or promote the fact that they sell hypodermic needles and syringes. Many pharmacy chains and independent pharmacies in these states follow these guidelines and legally sell hypodermic needles and syringes. In some states, only 10 needle/syringe combinations may be sold to an individual at a time, though the majority of states do not have this restriction.

What Would You Do?

While you are dispensing a drug product, you hear that a client has asked the pharmacist if he can purchase a dozen hypodermic needles and syringes. The client claims he is a diabetic. You know this client personally, and are sure of his illegal drug use in the past. What would you do in this scenario?

COMPOUNDING

Both state and federal law regulates the practice of **pharmacy compounding**. Currently, the Supreme Court has ruled that advertising of compounding services cannot be prohibited because this would violate rights to commercial free speech. The FDA has stepped in regarding cases of community pharmacies compounding certain drugs that are available in commercial preparations. Previously, pharmacists often compounded drug products without being required to have an NDA (new drug approval) from the FDA. The administration stated that this practice created "unapproved compounds" that could be dangerous. Pharmacists cannot advertise compounding services if they are compounding drug products that are otherwise commercially available in approved compounded products that have an NDA on file.

Much litigation between consumer groups and governmental bodies has occurred since the FDA became more focused on the compounding activities of pharmacists. As a result, pharmacists must follow their state laws as well as the FDA's guidelines concerning compounding very closely. Compounding outside of these guidelines may bring legal complications on either state or federal levels. Regardless, the issue of compounding is one that will see continued focus and revision as new medications are brought into the market. The roles of pharmacy technicians will be affected as new laws concerning compounding, and those individuals who are allowed to participate, are developed and amended. Pharmacy technicians will most likely see an increase in their approved duties in assisting pharmacists in compounding a variety of medications.

The United States Pharmacopoeia (USP) has consistently updated sterile compounding regulations. The USP <797> is an enforceable set of standards for nonsterile compounding, and provides a voluntary system of accreditation of compounding pharmacies. The USP <797> focus on enforceable standards for sterile compounding procedures and requirements. USP <797> has been adopted or enforced by the FDA, the Joint Commission, and also by various state boards of pharmacy. Because certain dosages that may be required are not available, or combinations of certain medications are not available, licensed pharmacists can compound these needed mixtures, though under strict regulations. Part of these regulations includes the level of "clean area" being used for compounding. The USP guidelines cover retail, hospital, and even home health-care compounding. The main goals of the continually improving regulation are to reduce contamination potential and keep unwanted particles in the air from infiltrating the compounded mixtures. Continuing education in compounding is required so that pharmacy workers are up-to-date. It is important to note that extemporaneous compounding of, for example, ointments for topical administration does not require the same level of sterility as do eye drops and intravenous medications.

The USP requires the following to protect compounded mixtures, the patients who receive them, and the pharmacy workers who compound them:

- For sterile compounding of eye drops and parenterals, barrier isolators that use positive pressure to keep airflow from less sterile areas into more sterile areas should be in place

- For sterile compounding of eye drops and parenterals, buffer areas or "ante rooms" that still must maintain certain "clean" levels; they are used for putting on and removing protective garb and equipment, and for disinfection of equipment

- Clean room areas for compounding of eye drops and parenterals, with a minimum of an ISO Class 7 rating, diluted airflow, temperature control, and humidity control; they must have specific materials on their ceilings, walls, and floors

- Gowning for compounding of eye drops and parenterals – including gloves, gowns or coats, hair covers, masks, shoe covers, and personal protective equipment as required

- Sterile products that must be used constantly and kept in the sterile area at all times

The Pharmacy Compounding Accreditation Board (PCAB) was formed to provide quality compounding standards through a voluntary pharmacy accreditation program. When the PCAB approves a pharmacy for accreditation, their seal of accreditation provides evidence that the pharmacy adheres to specific compounding standards and practices.

STATE REGULATION OF LONG-TERM CARE

Both state and federal law regulate certain components of long-term care. The licensing of the operators of long-term care pharmacies is licensed by state law in most cases. Certain states require pharmacists to have a more specialized license to practice in a long-term care pharmacy. Attaining long-term care licenses requires specific continuing education that focuses on long-term care pharmacies. When controlled substances are dispensed in a long-term care facility, the possibility of theft or sharing is increased due to the close proximity of patients with other patients, as well as the facility's staff members. The state looks closely at the operation of these facilities and the amounts of medications that the pharmacist dispenses because of the potential for misuse. Pharmacists must make sure that their understanding and continuing education about state regulations concerning long-term care is complete and current.

SUMMARY

State laws, in conjunction with the state boards of pharmacy, regulate pharmacy practice on a daily basis. The position of each state regarding its pharmacy regulations can be found in the tables published by the National Association of Boards of Pharmacy (NABP). Pharmacies, like other workplaces, must confirm to minimum OSHA requirements to provide a healthy and safe environment for employees.

Pharmacists must counsel patients exclusively – pharmacy technicians are not allowed to do this. However, pharmacy technicians can greatly help pharmacists by monitoring patient prescriptions, and checking for refills that seem to be requested more frequently than is normal. Controlled substance prescriptions can now be faxed in most states, but pharmacy technician and pharmacist monitoring of these is critical to prevent misuse and medication errors. Good patient record keeping is vital to ensure proper documentation of drug therapy, and for review of allergies, reactions, diseases, and conditions.

The ultimate goal of state laws concerning pharmacy practice is to provide quality therapeutic care, and to prevent patient harm. Pharmacists must remember that they have the ultimate responsibility for the patient's health. Pharmacy technicians must remember that there are more regulations today than ever before, which can affect their careers – a complete understanding of state laws and strict ethical practice is required. Compounding of medications is controlled by state and federal laws, with the FDA constantly monitoring the compounding activities of pharmacies. Because of increased regulation, pharmacy technicians will see an increase in their approved duties in assisting pharmacists.

SETTING THE SCENE

The following discussion and responses relate to the opening "Setting the Scene" scenario:

- The pharmacist should have consulted with the patient to explain the medication and all details.

- The pharmacist is in violation of the law because consultation with all Medicaid (and Medicare) patients is required.

- The pharmacist has the ultimate responsibility for patient care.

REVIEW QUESTIONS

Multiple Choice

1. The rules of pharmacy practice are set forth by which of the following agencies?

   A. National Association of Boards of Pharmacy
   B. Food and Drug Administration
   C. State Board of Pharmacy
   D. Drug Enforcement Agency

2. All of the following components are required on a prescription label, except:

   A. dispensing date
   B. address of the dispensing pharmacy
   C. any special third-party payer
   D. any federal or state cautions

3. Who must make decisions about patient refills if a hospital's automated computer system is not properly operational, or is experiencing "down time?"

   A. nurses
   B. pharmacists
   C. pharmacy technicians
   D. none of the above

4. Pharmacy technicians must make sure that the prescription information in the computer matches which of the following?

   A. the printed labels
   B. the fax numbers
   C. the prescription
   D. the USP

5. Practitioners who prescribe controlled substances must be registered with:

   A. OSHA
   B. DEA
   C. FDA
   D. NABP

6. Some states allow that needles and syringes can be legally purchased without a prescription if the patient is:

   A. over 18 years of age
   B. under 18 years of age
   C. a U.S. citizen
   D. none of the above

7. All drug products must be properly labeled and conform to the requirements of which of the following?

   A. Drug Enforcement Administration
   B. State Health Department
   C. State Board of Pharmacy
   D. all of the above

8. According to state law, when a prescription is submitted to a pharmacy for processing, the pharmacy technician must do all of the following, except:

   A. verify all of the information in the prescription is complete and clear
   B. translate the prescription information for the practitioner
   C. enter the prescription information into the computer system
   D. fill the prescription and have the pharmacist verify that it is correct, and packaged according to the standards of the pharmacy and state law

9. Pharmacy technicians should check the stock bottle's labeling and the National Drug Code number in the computer system; these should be compared to the original prescription. A good step to follow upon first use of the contents of the stock bottle is to mark its front label with which of the following letters?

   A. Z
   B. W
   C. X
   D. C

10. Faxed prescriptions for Schedule II drugs must be followed up by a written prescription, which must be received by the pharmacy within:

    A. 1 day
    B. 2 days
    C. 3 days
    D. 7 days

11. Prescriptions that are faxed and received on machines using fax paper must be immediately:

    A. dispensed to the patient
    B. photocopied and filed
    C. recorded into the pharmacy's computer system
    D. translated into English

12. Each pharmacy should make sure that every patient's record shows his or her entire available drug history, for at least:

    A. 1 year
    B. 2 years
    C. 3 years
    D. 5 years

13. While most states allow pharmacies to sell hypodermic needles and syringes in any quantity, there are some states that allow pharmacies to sell no more than:

    A. three at a time
    B. five at a time
    C. ten at a time
    D. two dozen at a time

14. A product identifier used for drugs intended for human use is called a:

    A. National Drug Code number
    B. Drug Enforcement Agency number
    C. United States Pharmacopoeia number
    D. Food and Drug Administration number

15. The state monitors the operation of long-term care facilities and the amount of medication that the pharmacist or technician dispenses because of:

    A. the potential for misuse
    B. the potential for addiction
    C. the price and cost of the medication
    D. all of the above

Fill in the Blank

1. A number (made up of alpha-numeric characters) assigned to a health-care practitioner that allows him or her to write prescriptions for controlled substances is called a _____.

2. Pharmacy technicians must understand both the laws of their state and _____ laws that regulate the practice of pharmacy.

3. Tables of information that enable pharmacists and pharmacy technicians to quickly find their state's position on a variety of pharmacy-related activities were created by the _____.

4. Unprofessional conduct must be _____ to the proper _____, as directed by the State Board of Pharmacy.

5. Computer dispensing systems can interact with robotic dispensing equipment to instruct the machinery which _____ are needed to be dispensed.

6. Most states now allow that controlled substance prescriptions can be _____.

7. A good amount of cost savings can be attained by the substitution of _____ drugs for _____ drugs.

8. The patient record should contain his or her full name, address, and _____ number.

9. Patient allergies must always be verified to avoid _____.

10. Computer systems used for pharmacy record keeping must have secure _____ systems in place in case the primary system becomes compromised or unable to be accessed.

CASE STUDY

Hillary, a certified pharmacy technician, dispensed a prescription for a patient. Jeremy, the pharmacist, knew that the prescriber's licensed was revoked the previous month.

1. What should Hillary have done before dispensing this medication?

2. What steps should Hillary take to examine the prescription to prevent forgeries?

3. What should the pharmacist ask the patient about the prescription?

RELATED INTERNET SITES

http://cr.pennnet.com

http://www.drugpolicy.org

http://www.drugsafetyinstitute.com

http://www.fda.gov

http://www.medscape.com

http://www.microcln.com

http://www.ncpanet.org

http://www.ncsl.org

http://www.pharmacytimes.com

http://www.uspharmacist.com

REFERENCES

Abood, R. (2005). *Pharmacy Practice and the Law* (4th ed.). Jones and Bartlett.

Fink, J. L., Vivian, J. C., & Bernstein, I. B. (2006). *Pharmacy Law Digest* (40th ed.). Wolters Kluwer Health.

Moini, J. (2005). *The Pharmacy Technician – A Comprehensive Approach.* Thomson/Delmar Learning.

University of the Sciences in Philadelphia (Ed.). (2008). *Remington: The Science and Practice of Pharmacy* (21st ed.). Lippincott Williams & Wilkins.

State Boards of Pharmacy

OBJECTIVES

Upon completion of this chapter, the reader should be able to:

1. Describe the Board of Pharmacy.
2. List the roles and responsibilities of the Board.
3. Describe the purpose of a state Board of Pharmacy.
4. Explain the enforcement powers of the Board of Pharmacy.
5. Define the major responsibilities of a state Board of Pharmacy.
6. Describe the Joint Commission and its responsibility regarding the pharmacy and the pharmacist.
7. Discuss pharmacist licensure renewal.
8. Describe disciplinary action against any pharmacist.
9. Explain pharmacy technician liability.
10. Identify the requirements for pharmacy licensure.

KEY TERMS

Continuing education – Instructional learning that keeps an individual up-to-date with advancements in their field.

Infringements – Violations of laws, regulations, or agreements.

Licensure – The practice of granting professional licenses to practice a profession.

Magistrates – Civil officers with the power to enforce laws.

National Formulary (NF) standards – Standards concerning medicines, dosage forms, drug substances, excipients (inactive substances used as carriers for active medicinal ingredients), medical devices, and dietary supplements.

Pharmacy internship – A period of service in a pharmacy, wherein a pharmacy student works, under supervision, to gain practical experience.

Prosecution – A legal proceeding against an individual.

Revocation – Recall of authority or power to act.

Revoked – Voided, annulled, recalled, withdrawn, or reversed.

United States Pharmacopoeia (USP) – The officially recognized authority and standard on the prescription of drugs, chemicals, and medicinal preparations in the United States.

SETTING THE SCENE

Jeff, a licensed hospital pharmacist, is on the phone, talking with a physician. After the phone call, the pharmacy technician, Jackie, tells Jeff that there are two men waiting to see him. They are inspectors from the Board of Pharmacy who wish to conduct an inspection.

Critical Thinking

- What would be the most common items found in the pharmacy that the inspectors would wish to investigate?

- If the pharmacist's license is expired, what would be the consequences?

- If the inspectors found that the locking mechanism on the door to the storage area for controlled substances was broken and could not be locked, what could be the penalty?

OVERVIEW

The regulation of the practice of pharmacy is primarily a state function and not a function of the federal government. The legal responsibilities of pharmacies vary from state to state. To provide better uniformity of state regulations, the National Association of Boards of Pharmacy (NABP) published a book entitled ***Model Rules for Pharmaceutical Care***. However, states may enact laws and Board of Pharmacy rules independent of the federal government, as long as they do not conflict with federal law. While pharmacy laws of the different states do vary, they agree with the fundamental principles, purposes, aims, and objectives of pharmacy practice. State Boards of Pharmacy also issue licenses for retail, hospital, and other types of pharmacies.

No one may practice pharmacy without a license unless he or she is licensed according to state law. Individuals may achieve such licensure by successfully completing the qualifications that their state has established. In most states, the Board of Pharmacy can take disciplinary action against any pharmacist or pharmacy, but each state has different approaches to how pharmacy technicians are regulated. Today, more states than ever before require that pharmacy technicians become certified before they are allowed to work in the pharmacy setting.

THE BOARD OF PHARMACY

The state Board of Pharmacy in each state is provided for by state laws (pharmacy practice acts). These boards strive to protect the health, safety, and welfare of the public. They are mostly made up of a combination of pharmacists, consumers, and health-care professionals. State Boards of Pharmacy are usually appointed by the governor of the state.

STATE BOARD OF PHARMACY'S FUNCTIONS

The Board of Pharmacy is a sub-agency that exists as part of a larger state agency, such as the Department of Health or Licensing. The Board of Pharmacy is charged with the enforcement and administration of pharmacy practice laws. This agency has powers delegated by the legislature via pharmacy practice statutes to put into effect rules or regulations to implement the statutes. A certain amount of enforcement discretion is vested by the Board of Pharmacy. While the Board is authorized to make rules and regulations for the enforcement and administration of pharmacy law, they must do so according to the expressed or implied purposes of the law.

The Board is an administrative agency, and not a legislative one. It may not exercise any power or authority that has not been clearly delegated to it. The Board of Pharmacy will grant licenses to qualified pharmacists, pharmacies, technicians, and interns. It also has the power to impose sanctions against those who do not follow all applicable laws. Licensure or registration may be canceled, **revoked** (withdrawn), or suspended according to conditions specified in certain statutes or regulations. Likewise, offenders may be placed on probation by the Board.

Many Boards of Pharmacy have other disciplinary sanctions available. These include civil fines and the imposing of a community services requirement. Some state laws specify that violations of the pharmacy act are punishable as criminal misdemeanors.

Drug distribution within a state is regulated by that state's Board of Pharmacy, which controls the practice of pharmacy for the protection of public health, safety, and welfare. It accomplishes this with rules and regulations. When these rules and regulations are violated, such action constitutes grounds for refusal, suspension, or **revocation** of any license or permit issued.

The Board may also conduct hearings or proceedings to revoke, suspend, or refuse renewal of any license or permit issued under the authority of the pharmacy act. The Board of Pharmacy assists state law enforcement agencies in enforcing all laws that pertain to drugs, narcotics, and pharmacy practice.

Most states issue licensure permits for pharmacy practice that last 1 to 2 years. Pharmacists must be periodically relicensed. Certificates of licensure must always be prominently displayed at the pharmacy. Pharmacists who are licensed in one state may obtain licensure in another state without taking another full licensure examination. However, as discussed elsewhere in this chapter, some states do not accept Florida licensure and require examinations for people moving to their state from Florida.

The many new areas of pharmacy practice are greatly affecting its regulation. These new areas include clinical pharmacy, nuclear pharmacy (a pharmacy which provides radiopharmaceutical services), mandated counseling, drug-product selection, and pharmaceutical care. Many states have adopted provisions that were initially set forth in the National Association of Boards of Pharmacy (NABP)'s *Model State Pharmacy Practice Act (MSPPA)*. A copy of this act may be viewed online at http://www.nabp.net.

ENFORCEMENT POWERS

Most situations wherein the Board of Pharmacy can institute actions involve those that are civil in nature. Their powers may also include those of arrest (when a felony is committed in the presence of an enforcement officer), though warrants for arrest are issued by magistrates or judges. In criminal cases, the Board conducts investigations and turns over evidence to state or county prosecutors. The FDA and DEA enforce federal drug laws by investigating matters and turning them over to the U.S. Attorney's office for prosecution.

Boards of Pharmacy can enforce statutes, state drug control acts, and their own regulations by suspension, revocation, or withholding of licenses or permits, by monetary penalties, or by seeking court injunctions, restraining orders, or other court orders. They may also refuse to renew a pharmacist's license or a pharmacy's permit due to infringements. State Boards of Pharmacy are responsible for all of the following:

1. Licensing by examination or license transfer – State Boards of Pharmacy are responsible for granting pharmacist licenses and pharmacy technician certificates. They accomplish this by holding examinations, such as the NAPLEX, that must be passed in order for an individual to practice. They also transfer licenses that existed in other states so that an individual can practice in a new location. During this process, the background of each applicant is thoroughly checked. In some states, pharmacy technicians must be registered to practice.

2. Renewal of licenses – In most states, licenses are granted for 2 years. Renewal of licenses can occur after an individual has applied for renewal on a timely basis, and completed continuing education since the previous licensure. After review,

the state Board of Pharmacy determines if the individual has met all necessary requirements in order to have his or her license renewed. Other states simply require the individual to update all of his or her information on file and pay the renewal fee. Some pharmacists can even renew their licenses via the Internet (in certain states).

3. Establishment and enforcement of compliance in pharmacy practice – State Boards of Pharmacy assess penalties against those who violate their regulations of practice. They establish standards of behavior that must be followed by pharmacy technicians and pharmacists alike. Penalties include fines, revocation, or suspension of pharmacist licenses, legal actions, and even imprisonment in severe cases.

4. Approval of degree programs to teach the practice of pharmacy – State Boards of Pharmacy offer accreditation for pharmacy degree programs offered by colleges and universities. These programs are rigidly controlled so that each school conforms to the requirements of the Board of Pharmacy in its state. State laws also uniformly allow state Boards of Pharmacy to recognize national accreditation, under the ACPE regulation through the U.S. No state accredits specific pharmacy schools.

5. The suspension, revocation, or restriction of pharmacy licenses – State Boards of Pharmacy review individual cases and can determine that an applicant's license may need to be suspended, revoked, or even restricted. Suspension of a pharmacy license means that it is placed "on hold" for a specific period while the individual or company fulfills the requirements of the state board, after which the license will be reactivated. Revocation of a license means that the license has been nullified by the state board and cannot be reactivated. Restriction of a license means that the individual or company may continue to practice, but only within certain parameters allowed by the state board; certain activities are allowed, while others are not.

6. Control of the training, qualifications, and employment of pharmacy personnel – The state Boards of Pharmacy monitor the quality of pharmacies and their personnel, requiring specialized training that is of a certain approved level. Unqualified or untrained personnel cannot legally practice until they fulfill these requirements. Pharmacies can only employ properly qualified and trained personnel, including pharmacy technicians.

7. The collection of demographic data – State Boards of Pharmacy collect demographic data about the staff members of

each pharmacy in their jurisdiction. This information may be provided by the state boards to specific governmental bodies in order to assess the overall practice of pharmacy in each state.

8. The right to seize drugs and devices that may cause harm to the public – Upon discovery of a drug or device that has the potential to harm the public, the state Boards of Pharmacy may seize the item(s) and make a decision about their continued use. These items include medications, medical devices, and peripheral equipment that relates to drugs and therapies.

9. Establishing specifications for pharmacy facilities and equipment – State Boards of Pharmacy control the types of facilities required by each pharmacy, as well as the equipment that can be used within. All items used in the pharmacy setting must conform to the state Board of Pharmacy's listings of approved equipment. Each state has its own specifications for pharmacy facilities and equipment.

10. Establishing standards for purity and quality – The state Board of Pharmacy in each state establishes purity and quality standards for compounding, which may be further regulated by federal standards. Usually, the more restrictive standard (be it state or federal) prevails when there is a discrepancy.

11. The issuance and renewal of licenses related to manufacturing and distribution of pharmaceutical drugs and devices – State Boards of Pharmacy issue and renew licenses to pharmaceutical manufacturers and distributors, as regulated by the FDA. Severe penalties exist if these companies do not fully adhere to the guidelines of the state. Individualized regulations apply to both prescription and OTC drugs and devices.

12. Inspection of pharmacy personnel, facilities, and equipment – State Boards of Pharmacy may conduct unannounced inspections of pharmacies, paying attention to the facilities themselves, the equipment they use on a regular basis, and even the personnel within. They may check for proper display of licenses, conditions of the workplace, potential hazards, improper storage of medications, medical devices, and other equipment, and even question pharmacy staff members about their daily job duties.

13. Establishing standards for the integrity and confidentiality of patient information – The private health information of patients requires protection. This is accomplished by the state Boards of Pharmacy and the regulations and standards they establish concerning the integrity and confidentiality of the

information. Those who violate PHI confidentiality standards may face severe penalties, with the most serious penalties given for intentional misuse of PHI. Those who unintentionally misuse PHI may receive minor penalties intended to correct their future behavior while still allowing them to practice and increase their knowledge of pharmacy.

What Would You Do?

Sean has been working in a retail pharmacy for 10 years. His certification expires and he must renew it quickly in order to continue to practice. If you were Sean, what must you do to renew your certification?

EXAMINATION REQUIREMENTS

Applicants for a pharmacist license must pass all of the following, within differing periods of time per state law, after graduating from a state-approved school of pharmacy:

- Part I – North American Pharmacist Licensing Exam (NAPLEX)
- Part II – Multi-state Pharmacy Jurisprudence Exam (MPJE)
- Part III – Written and Practical (Compounding) Exam – however, only 10 states currently require Part III

For the NAPLEX, applicants must submit a completed licensure application and have their completed education documentation approved before they are allowed to take the exam. Once approved, they can apply to take the exam online at http://www.nabp.net. In addition, some states require applicants to have their college or school submit a tentative graduation date to the NABP, plus "Form 2 – Certification of Professional Education" with an official education transcript.

Focus On...

NAPLEX

As of 2008, all states now use the North American Pharmacist Licensing Exam (NAPLEX).

For the MPJE, the same requirements exist, plus applicants must have their completed internship experience submitted and approved. For the Written and Practical (Compounding) Exam, applicants must meet all requirements for the MPJE.

INTERNSHIP REQUIREMENTS

Most states require pharmacy internships to last between 400 and 2,500 hours, based on 40 hours per week, working under the supervision of a licensed pharmacist. Special projects are often required during these internships, and performance standards must be constantly met. Internships are usually completed both while the student is still actively attending courses, and after schooling is completed, but prior to licensure.

The term **pharmacy internship** means "supervised practical experience working under a licensed pharmacist's direction." The purpose of a pharmacy internship program is to acquire the knowledge and practical experience that is necessary to function competently and effectively upon licensure. The supervising pharmacist must submit proof of an intern's completion of required clock hours on a *practical experience affidavit*.

During a pharmacy internship, interns will receive comprehensive instruction and experience in these (and possibly other) important areas of pharmacy practice:

1. Receiving and interpreting prescriptions and medication orders
2. Compounding prescriptions and medication orders
3. Dispensing prescriptions and medication orders
4. Reviewing patient medication profiles
5. Communicating with patients
6. Consulting with other health-care professionals
7. Managing the pharmacy

LICENSURE OF THE PHARMACIST

State Boards of Pharmacy issue licenses to pharmacists and pharmacies. The National Association of Boards of Pharmacy (NABP) represents state pharmaceutical licensing authorities. All states have standards dealing with pharmacy practices. In order to become a licensed pharmacist, most states require each applicant to:

- have graduated from an *accredited* school of pharmacy
- have completed a required internship
- have passed the state's pharmacy licensure exam
- have a documentable history of good moral character

Ten states require pharmacists to be 21 or older, with most of the rest requiring pharmacists to be at least 18 years of age.

Each pharmacy location is issued a separate license by its state Board of Pharmacy. Some states grant licensure by transfer from another jurisdiction (reciprocity), though many states do not allow reciprocity based on a Florida license. These states include Arkansas, Connecticut, Georgia, Hawaii, Idaho, Louisiana, Minnesota, Ohio, Oklahoma, Tennessee, West Virginia, and Wyoming. Florida itself only allows reciprocity if the NAPLEX exam was taken within the prior 12 years. California only allows reciprocity if the applicant took the NAPLEX after 2004.

While some states do not regulate who can actually own a pharmacy, some states do not allow physicians to own pharmacies because of possible conflicts of interest. An example would be a physician's office referring its patients exclusively to the pharmacy that it owns.

Focus On...

Licensing of Pharmacists

Pharmacists may become licensed in most states by simply transferring their license from another state, depending on the states involved. In general, this removes the requirement of taking the Board of Pharmacy examination in a new state.

PHARMACIST LICENSURE RENEWAL

Periodically, pharmacists must renew their licenses by paying a fee and, in some states, by completing a certain number of continuing education credits. Renewal of a license usually requires the revealing of in-depth personal information, continuing education record forms, the pharmacy's permit information, verification of any disciplinary actions taken during the previous licensure period and explanation of outcomes, and the renewal fee.

Some states currently offer online renewal, which can expedite the process. All states require completely correct filing of paperwork or online renewal information and usually will refuse to renew an applicant if anything is still incomplete at the end of the allowed renewal period.

Focus On...

Licensure Renewal

It is not the responsibility of the state Boards of Pharmacy to deliver a license renewal to a licensee. Instead, it is the responsibility of each pharmacist to seek out and obtain a licensure renewal.

CONTINUING EDUCATION REQUIREMENTS

Though the amount of credits and hours of continuing education vary per state, all states require continuing education as part of pharmacy practice and licensure. Continuing education credits may be completed in both formal courses given by approved providers, and in self-study courses. Appropriate subjects for pharmacy practitioners generally include, but are not limited to:

- Techniques for the reduction of medication and prescription errors
- Knowledge of drug interactions
- Pharmacology of new or developing drugs
- Infection control
- Reporting of suspected child abuse
- Public health issues
- Legal and regulatory issues (one hour of continuing education credits must now focus on pharmacy law)
- Proper patient counseling
- Sterile procedures

Approved providers of continuing education generally include:

- American Council on Pharmaceutical Education (ACPE)–approved sponsors or providers (this list is available at http://www.acpe-accredit.org)
- State Board of Pharmacy – approved sponsors or providers
- Colleges, universities, and other degree-granting institutions (these are usually listed under individual state Web sites, but the degrees they offer must include A.A.S., B.S., M.S., Pharm.D., or Ph.D. in Pharmacy)

STATE BOARD INSPECTIONS

Periodically, pharmacy board inspectors conduct routine inspections of pharmacies for compliance with various laws and regulations. These laws and regulations for pharmacy operation vary per state. All licensed personnel as well as appropriate records may be inspected, and employees are expected to cooperate with inspectors. Though most inspections are more educational than investigative, the pharmacist should be aware of any inspections that involve searches for incriminating evidence.

CERTIFICATION OF PHARMACY TECHNICIANS

States regulate pharmacy technician certification, and differ from each other in their requirements. To ensure that pharmacy technicians in every state have at least a minimum level of skill, the Pharmacy Technician Certification Board (PTCB) has been established. The overall goal of the PTCB is to improve the proficiency of pharmacy technicians in every state so that they may serve patients, co-workers, and pharmacists more competently.

The PTCB offers an examination called the Pharmacy Technician Certification Examination (PTCE) three times per year. This examination is divided into three areas of competence:

- Assisting the Pharmacist

- Maintenance of Medication/Inventory Control Systems

- Helping with Administration and Management of the Pharmacy

The examination includes questions that focus on drug names and classifications, federal pharmacy law, mathematics (as used in the pharmacy), and pharmacy operations. Certified pharmacy technicians may use the initials "*CPhT*" following their names. Pharmacies in some states pay certified pharmacy technicians higher wages than those who are not certified, though this is not yet true everywhere.

Renewal of pharmacy technician certification requires continuing education. In order to have his or her certification renewed, a pharmacy technician must complete 20 hours of continuing education credits every 2 years. Continuing education may be obtained at a variety of pharmacy seminars, through pharmacy organizations and journal publications, and even over the Internet. The individual requirements of each state are not the same, so it is important that pharmacy technicians verify what the state Board of Pharmacy requires them to do. Every year, more states are increasing their requirements for pharmacy technicians, and more are requiring that they become certified.

The other nationally accredited pharmacy technician certification exam is the ExCPT, which is given by the Institute for the Certification of Pharmacy Technicians (ICPT). The mission of the ICPT is to recognize pharmacy technicians who have the knowledge and skills needed to assist pharmacists to safely, accurately, and efficiently prepare and dispense prescriptions, and to promote high standards of practice. The ExCPT exam is available to all pharmacy technicians, regardless of the type of pharmacy in which they practice. The exam, which consists of 110 multiple-choice questions, certifies each applicant who passes for 2 years, after which recertification is required. To reinstate your certification, you must complete at least 20 hours of continuing education, 1 hour of which must be on pharmacy law.

Focus On...

State Certification, Registration, and Licensure Requirements

As of 2008, only seven states (Illinois, Indiana, Louisiana, Montana, Oregon, South Carolina, and Washington) require certification of pharmacy technicians, though negotiations in other states are ongoing. Most states (a total of 35) now require pharmacy technicians to be registered in order to practice. There are now eight states that require pharmacy technicians to obtain a license: Alaska, Arizona, California, Massachusetts, Oregon, Rhode Island, Utah, and Wyoming.

For the latest updates, go to http://www.nationaltechexam.org (under "ExCPT exam," click on "State by State Tech Requirements").

DRUG CONTROL REGULATIONS

Pharmacists who violate the federal Controlled Substances Act are handled according to whether they knowingly and intentionally violated the act. Unintentional violations, such as those related to bookkeeping, are punished with a civil (not criminal) penalty. Harsher penalties await those who knowingly and intentionally violate the act, with criminal adjudication occurring commonly. Federal or state violations involving controlled substances can have severe implications on a pharmacist's licensure and can even keep him or her from practicing pharmacy at all in the future.

HOSPITAL PHARMACY

The state regulation of hospital pharmacy is quite different from the regulation of community pharmacy. Areas of difference that have prompted new hospital pharmacy regulation include in-hospital dispensing of drugs, the licensure of hospital pharmacy personnel, and the appropriate functions of the hospital pharmacy technician. The PTCB has unique state-by-state regulations for pharmacy technicians working in hospital or institutional pharmacies. In general, pharmacy technicians in most of these pharmacies are not allowed to accept called-in prescriptions from physicians, check the work of other pharmacy technicians, or transfer prescription orders. However, they are allowed to enter prescriptions into the pharmacy computer system and compound medications for dispensing. Also, many states require that directors of hospital pharmacies possess special training or expertise.

REGULATION OF LONG-TERM CARE PHARMACIES

Under current legislation, long-term care facilities may be separately licensed under state law. Pharmacists in these facilities are usually required by state law to have special training or expertise, and must complete individualized continuing education in order to recertify their licenses. Pharmacists must be very careful to correctly dispense medications in these facilities under the full approval of their state laws. The rules are still in force about the use of strong (often Schedule II) medications even though the patient resides in a long-term care facility and may need these medications until the end of his or her life. The long-term care pharmacist supervises all aspects of the drugs required by residents of these facilities, as regulated by the laws of their state and OBRA drug review requirements. He or she must maintain strict drug control, regular drug regimen reviews, cost controls, review committees, and detailed pharmacy policies and procedures. Techniques such as personal patient supervision and infusion therapy teams help to control medication use. Comprehensive medication reviews help to identify and prevent adverse outcomes.

STANDARDS OF THE JOINT COMMISSION

The Joint Commission sets certain voluntary standards for hospitals and provides accreditation based on their compliance with Joint Commission standards. These standards are important, serving as a guide to the proper method of operating a hospital, ensuring competence, licensure, controls, records, accuracy, and evaluation. Though the Joint Commission standards are voluntary, not being accredited by them is detrimental to a hospital's survival, as many insurance companies will not pay a non-accredited hospital. There are six basic Joint Commission standards:

1. The hospital pharmacy must be staffed with competent, legally qualified personnel, with a pharmacist available at all times on duty, on call, or as a consultant. Non-pharmacist personnel must be assigned only duties that are consistent with their training. Clerical services must be provided. The pharmacy must be licensed as required. If there is no pharmacy at the hospital, pharmaceutical services must be obtained from another hospital pharmacy.

2. Drugs for external use only must be separated from drugs for internal use only and stored and controlled in accordance

with the United States Pharmacopoeia (USP) and National Formulary (NF) standards (see Appendix G). Provisions must be made for emergency drugs on carts or in kits. The metric system must be used for all medications. Conversion charts must be made available.

3. Adequate record keeping systems and procedural guidelines for pharmaceutical preparation must be developed. Pharmacy personnel must participate in applicable patient care programs. Patient medication profiles should be maintained and reviewed for potential drug interactions. Patients must be instructed in correct drug use.

4. The pharmacist must review inpatient drug orders before initial dosage dispensation except in an emergency. There must be proper drug recall procedures. Drug defects must be reported to the USP/FDA drug defect program. Proper labeling of inpatient and outpatient medications must be initiated. Outpatient labels must contain the pharmacy's name, address, and phone number; the date; the drug's serial number; the patient's full name; the drug's name, strength, and amount dispensed; patient directions; the name or initials of the dispensing individual; and any required cautionary labeling.

5. There must be automatic cancellation of standing orders when a patient goes to surgery. A system of drug stop orders must be in existence. Identification of each patient before drug administration must be made. Abbreviations when ordering drugs must be discouraged. Drugs must be ordered by a practitioner and properly labeled when given to a patient upon discharge.

6. The pharmacy's activities must be monitored and evaluated in accordance with the hospital's quality assurance program.

You Be the Judge

Betty, a pharmacy technician, is working in a hospital pharmacy. While she is repacking drugs, she discovers that some of them have defective packaging. However, she ignores this and repacks the drugs anyway. What do you think that Betty should have done in this case?

DISCIPLINARY ACTION

In most states, the Board of Pharmacy can take disciplinary action against any pharmacist if they have proof of the following:

1. The pharmacist's license was obtained through fraud, misrepresentation, or deceit

2. The pharmacist has been determined to be mentally incompetent

3. The pharmacist has knowingly violated or allowed the violation of any state or federal provision or law, rule, or regulation concerning drug possession, use, distribution, or dispensation

4. The pharmacist has knowingly allowed an unlicensed or unauthorized person to run the pharmacy or engage in the practice of pharmacy

5. The pharmacist has compounded, dispensed, or caused the compounding or dispensing of any drug or device containing a quantity of ingredients other than that required by law

You Be the Judge

Karen is a pharmacist who has been practicing at a retail pharmacy in Miami, Florida. Recently, the state Board of Pharmacy revoked her license. She is planning to move to the state of New York within a short period of time. What do you think that Karen is required to do in this case in order to practice pharmacy in New York?

STATUS OF PHARMACY TECHNICIANS

Every pharmacy technician should know and understand the regulations of his or her state Board of Pharmacy. In order to practice as a pharmacy technician, some states require pharmacy technicians to be registered. Their status must be maintained continually by completing continuing education requirements as set forth by the state Board of Pharmacy. All statutes, be they state or federal, must be continually obeyed. Regulations concerning the status of pharmacy technicians differ amongst the states. As the duties of pharmacy technicians have been expanding because of the growth of the pharmacy industry, regulatory changes in what they can and cannot legally do have followed. Each state has different approaches in how pharmacy technicians are regulated. More states than ever before require that pharmacy technicians become certified before being allowed to work in the pharmacy setting.

Traditional pharmacy technician activities include, but are not limited to:

• Accepting written prescriptions

• Checking prescriptions for accuracy and completeness

• Creating patient profiles

- Determining patient benefit plan information
- Retrieving patient profiles
- Entering prescription information on patient profiles
- Obtaining drug products to use in filling prescriptions
- Counting numbers of tablets and other drug forms
- Manually filling prescriptions
- Using appropriately sized containers

Many states now allow pharmacy technicians to call physicians for refill authorization. Few states allow pharmacy technicians to accept new called-in prescriptions from a physician's office, and those that do have instituted many regulations concerning this practice. One area of extreme change is in the allowing of pharmacy technicians to reconstitute oral liquids. Other newer areas of pharmacy technician duties include managing new automated technology, implementing or revising policies and procedure manuals, and training other technicians by providing in-service and other types of training programs.

Focus On...

Pharmacy Technicians

The pharmacist on duty is responsible for the supervision of non-pharmacist support personnel. This particularly applies to the supervision of pharmacy technicians.

PHARMACY TECHNICIANS IN RETAIL SETTINGS

About 7 out of 10 pharmacy technician jobs are in retail settings, which may be either independently owned or part of a chain. These settings may be in dedicated pharmacies, or as part of drug stores, grocery stores, department stores, or mass retailers. An increasing number of job openings are resulting from the expansion of retail pharmacies and similar settings, and from the need to replace workers who change occupations or leave the labor force.

As the population grows and ages, demand for pharmaceuticals, and therefore the trained individuals required for their preparation and dispensation, will increase dramatically. Because of growth, pharmacist-to-technician ratios have changed in many states. It is common for a pharmacist to supervise three or more pharmacy technicians in today's pharmacy practice. Many retail pharmacies are now open 24 hours, requiring pharmacists and pharmacy technicians to work varying shifts, also leading to more employment opportunities.

PHARMACY TECHNICIANS IN HOSPITAL SETTINGS

About 2 out of 10 pharmacy technician jobs are in hospital settings. In the hospital, pharmacy technicians (in most states) are responsible for the following:

- Unit dose and other medication preparation
- Checking patient charts in conjunction with prescriptions
- Preparing, packaging, and labeling medications
- Delivering medications to nurses
- Managing robotic stocking systems
- Organizing 24-hour supplies of medications for all patients
- Cataloguing information in the hospital computer system

Focus On...

State Boards of Pharmacy
Each state Board of Pharmacy regulates the roles, duties, and expectations of pharmacy technicians who practice in the state.

PHARMACY TECHNICIANS' LIABILITIES

Most states require that a pharmacy technician must work under the close, direct observation of a licensed pharmacist. Usually, the supervising pharmacist is responsible for any negligence committed by the pharmacy technician. As technicians take over an increasing proportion of drug dispensing functions, their opportunities to be involved in medication errors increase.

Other common areas wherein pharmacy technicians may be liable include:

- not advising the pharmacist of known drug interactions
- providing incorrect information to patients
- providing advice to patients when the state does not allow them to do so

Pharmacy technicians may be suspended from work, be fined, be fired, and even receive jail sentences depending on their negligent or criminal actions. Though pharmacists have the utmost authority over and responsibility for the actions of their pharmacy technicians, the technicians themselves can be in serious legal trouble if their duties are not conducted properly at all times. Liability insurance is available for pharmacy technicians, and it is recommended that they purchase it in order to protect themselves. It is important to always remember that patients' lives hang in the balance.

Focus On...

Disciplinary Action

State Boards of Pharmacy have the authority to discipline pharmacy technicians for improper behavior.

SUMMARY

Pharmacists must attend a pharmacy school as well as pass rigorous examinations in order to be able to obtain licensure. Pharmacy internships are also required to ensure that pharmacists have plenty of experience in the pharmacy setting before being allowed to practice on their own. Once they are ready, pharmacists obtain their licenses to practice from the state in which they will work. Continuing education credits are required in all states so that pharmacists are continually learning about their field, ensuring better patient care. Disciplinary action can be taken by the state Board of Pharmacy against pharmacists who violate regulations of practice. Likewise, as pharmacy technicians are allowed to handle many of the duties traditionally handled by pharmacists, regulatory control of their activities is on the rise. Pharmacy technicians must receive specialized training in the areas of pharmacy in which they will work, be it in the community setting, the hospital, or in other settings.

In all states, the Board of Pharmacy can discipline pharmacists and pharmacy technicians if they violate state or federal laws. Each state has its own regulations concerning pharmacy technician certifications, and regulates pharmacy technicians in different ways. All states also require pharmacy technicians to work under close, direct observation of licensed pharmacists. These pharmacists are usually held responsible for any negligent acts of pharmacy technicians. Criminal and/or negligent actions by pharmacy technicians may result in suspension, termination, fines, and even imprisonment.

SETTING THE SCENE

The following discussion and responses relate to the opening "Setting the Scene" scenario:

- Pharmacy board inspectors commonly check all licensure documents of the pharmacy and its staff, as well as the pharmacy records.

- The inspectors will charge the pharmacist with "practicing without a license," which will lead to fines, continuing education hours that must be completed, and other penalties based on the length of time that the license has been expired.

- This is a potentially dangerous situation, because if access to the controlled substances area was not protected by a functioning lock, anyone could enter and take whatever substances they wanted. A fine would probably be the punishment for having a non-secured facility.

REVIEW QUESTIONS

Multiple Choice

1. All of the following are powers of the Board of Pharmacy, except:

    A. to regulate the practice of pharmacy
    B. to administer and enforce all laws placed under its jurisdiction
    C. to distribute drugs within the state
    D. to investigate violations of law under the pharmacy act itself

2. The pharmacy board may discipline a pharmacy that is in violation of the law by:

    A. firing the pharmacist
    B. not issuing a renewal of the pharmacy permit
    C. refusing funding for the pharmacy
    D. prosecuting the pharmacist through the U.S. Attorney General's office

3. State Boards of Pharmacy are responsible for:

   A. renewal of licenses
   B. approval of degree programs to teach the practice of pharmacy
   C. the establishment of standards for purity and quality
   D. all of the above

4. Which of the following organizations sets certain voluntary standards for hospitals?

   A. NABP
   B. FDA
   C. DEA
   D. the Joint Commission

5. The pharmacy department's activities must be monitored and evaluated in accordance with which of the following?

   A. the hospital's quality assurance program
   B. the hospital's pharmacy directors
   C. the hospital's vice president
   D. the FDA

6. Which of the following are the duties and responsibilities of the National Association of Boards of Pharmacy (NABP)?

   A. coordination of uniformity of the state Boards of Pharmacy
   B. controls scheduled drugs
   C. coordination of the DEA and FDA
   D. coordination of the CDC to prevent communicable diseases

7. State Boards of Pharmacy are responsible for all of the following, except:

   A. establishment and enforcement of compliance in pharmacy practice
   B. approval of degree programs to teach the practice of pharmacy
   C. establishing standards of college academia for pharmacy technicians
   D. inspection of pharmacy personnel, facilities, and equipment

8. According to the standards of the Joint Commission, non-pharmacist personnel must be assigned duties that are consistent with:

   A. their training
   B. staff shortages
   C. their skills
   D. the demands of nurses

9. Which of the following statements is *not* true regarding applying for pharmacist licensure?

   A. the applicant must have knowledge in medicine at the level of a practitioner
   B. the applicant must have graduated from an accredited pharmacy school or college
   C. the applicant must be above 18 years of age
   D. the applicant must have demonstrated a good moral character

10. A pharmacist may complete his continuing education in which of the following ways?

    A. formal courses
    B. self-training courses
    C. self-study courses
    D. A and C

11. Which of the following statements is required during pharmacist licensure renewal?

    A. completing a certain number of continuing education credits
    B. paying a fee
    C. verification of any disciplinary actions taken during the previous licensure period and explanation of outcomes
    D. all of the above

12. Which of the following currently allow(s) pharmacy technicians to call physicians for refill authorization?

    A. only the state of Florida
    B. the states of Florida and New York
    C. many states
    D. none of the above

13. Pharmacy technicians may be liable for which of the following areas?

    A. providing advice to patients
    B. providing patients' insurance information
    C. advising the pharmacist of known drug interactions
    D. advising coworkers about medication errors

14. Which of the following unintentional violations of the federal Controlled Substances Act is punished with a civil penalty?

    A. selling narcotic drugs
    B. purchasing non-narcotic drugs
    C. bookkeeping of controlled substances
    D. all of the above

15. Which of the following is *not* a responsibility of pharmacy technicians in the hospital setting?

    A. delivering medications to nurses
    B. preparing, packaging, and labeling drugs
    C. providing advice to nurses and patients
    D. checking patient charts in conjunction with prescriptions

Fill in the Blank

1. The Board of Pharmacy is a legislative body that has the authority to pass _____ regulations.

2. Many states have adopted provisions that were set forth by the National Association of _____.

3. In most states, the Board of Pharmacy can take disciplinary action against any pharmacist whose license was obtained through _____, misrepresentation, or deceit.

4. State Boards of Pharmacy are responsible for approval of degree programs to teach the practice of _____.

5. State Boards of Pharmacy are mostly made up of pharmacists, health-care professionals, and _____.

6. The pharmacist must review inpatient drug orders before initial dosage dispensation except in an_____.

CASE STUDY

A pharmacy technician practicing in the state of Oregon, which requires both active certification and licensure, remembers to recertify herself, but ignores renewing her license on time. After 2 months, the state Board of Pharmacy contacts her about her expired license.

1. What will this pharmacy technician have to do in order to become relicensed?

2. Which examination or examinations must she have taken in order to become relicensed?

3. How long does the license last until it expires again?

RELATED INTERNET SITES

http://careers.pharmacytimes.com

http://drugtopics.modernmedicine.com

http://www.bls.gov

http://www.jobpharm.com

http://www.jointcommission.org

http://www.medscape.com

http://www.nabp.net

http://www.nationaltechexam.org; **click on "State by State Tech Requirements" under "ExCPT exam"**

http://www.nhanow.com

http://www.pharmacychoice.com

http://www.ptcb.org

REFERENCES

Fink, J. L., Vivian, J. C., & Bernstein, I. B. (2006). *Pharmacy Law Digest* (40th ed.). Wolters Kluwer Health.

Moini, J. (2005). *The Pharmacy Technician – A Comprehensive Approach*. Thomson/Delmar Learning.

Reiss, B. S., & Hall, G. D. (2006). *Guide to Federal Pharmacy Law* (5th ed.). Apothecary Press.

Strandberg, K. M. (2002). *Essentials of Law and Ethics for Pharmacy Technicians*. CRC Press.

University of the Sciences in Philadelphia. (Ed.). (2008). *Remington: The Science and Practice of Pharmacy* (21st ed.). Lippincott Williams & Wilkins.

CHAPTER 1

What Would You Do?

Brian has had three traffic violations in the past three months. He has also been charged with domestic violence against his girlfriend. You are the pharmacist for whom Brian works, and you are aware of some of these events. One day, you hear him verbally provoking another worker until an argument breaks out. Brian becomes very agitated. Knowing his background, what would you do in this situation?

In this situation, it would be wise for the pharmacist to ask Brian to leave the pharmacy and take the rest of the day off. The next day, the situation should be discussed with Brian, and a letter written explaining that his behavior cannot be tolerated at work. This letter can serve as a legal notice to Brian that the pharmacy can terminate his employment should his adverse behavior continue.

You Be the Judge

Mark has been working in a retail pharmacy for 17 years. He is a senior technician, and a reliable person at work. About a year ago, his wife died, causing him to become very depressed. Last week, he made a mistake while he was compounding two medications. The pharmacist found out about his failure to exercise reasonable care while working. He told Mark that this was a case of negligence and that he could be charged for his error. Mark responded rudely and even pushed the pharmacist.

In your judgment, what would be the possible consequences for Mark, taking his entire situation into account? What could he be charged with for being physically violent with the pharmacist?

In this situation, since Mark has been a good employee and only recently had problems because of the death of his wife, it may be a good idea to suggest grief counseling to Mark. However, the pharmacist was correct about potential charges against Mark for negligence. If the pharmacist chose to press charges against Mark, he could be charged with felony battery, though it is unlikely since there was no actual injury to the pharmacist. Usually, Mark's actions against the pharmacist would be considered a misdemeanor, especially since there was no threat of a weapon being used.

You Be the Judge

Pamela is a pharmacy technician who recently dispensed eyedrops for a patient with glaucoma. The patient used the eyedrops per the enclosed instructions, but experienced no positive effects, and, after 1 week, continued experiencing minor but continuing visual impairment. The patient went back to her physician and complained about the eyedrops she had used. He checked the eyedrops, finding out that they were long past their expiration date. In your judgment, what would the possible consequences be for Pamela since the expiration date had not been checked before the medication was dispensed by the pharmacist? In addition, what would happen to the pharmacist because of this error?

Both Pamela and the pharmacist are responsible for not checking the expiration date; this product should have been removed from stock.

If the patient decides to sue, the pharmacist is legally responsible for negligence, and Pamela is responsible for negligence if causation can be proved—that her actions, in fact, caused a negative outcome for the patient. The pharmacist is legally responsible for the actions of the pharmacy technician, and could be fined or even have his license revoked.

CHAPTER 2

You Be the Judge

Phil is a pharmacy technician who is asked by a customer about Plan B®, which is intended for use as a morning-after pill. Because Phil believes that the use of a morning-after medication to prevent conception is wrong, he describes all sorts of serious adverse effects and states that they happen to *most* of the people who take the drug. As a result, the patient calls her doctor, who later calls the pharmacy and speaks with the pharmacist, telling him what Phil said and asking for an explanation. In your judgment, was Phil ethically correct in his actions? What sorts of legal repercussions do you think could await Phil as a result of his misstatements about Plan B?

Phil was not ethically correct in misrepresenting the facts about Plan B to the patient, and in the fact that he did not respect the patient's autonomy. He was not legally correct in advising this patient; he should have immediately referred her to the pharmacist. Because counseling a patient is outside the scope of a pharmacy technician's practice, he could lose his job as a result.

What Would You Do?

It is a busy afternoon, and the pharmacy has only one pharmacy technician on duty. The pharmacist does not consult with two patients because of all his other responsibilities, and they leave the pharmacy. If you were the pharmacist in this situation, what should you have done?

The pharmacist is ethically, morally, and legally responsible for consulting with patients. Consulting and supporting patients is more important than other activities—and this should have been given higher priority. A pharmacist's role as a patient advocate is of the utmost importance in preventing medication errors. It is important to prioritize in the pharmacy—with patient consultation being most important.

You Be the Judge

Molly, a young pharmacy technician, goes into work early Monday morning after spending Sunday night out late at a nightclub with her friends. She has a bad hangover. How could Molly's condition affect her ability to provide good patient care? What could Molly have done instead of coming to work in this condition? What may be the consequences of this type of behavior?

Molly's condition could impair her ability to make accurate judgments and concentrate on providing high-quality service to patients, potentially making errors that could harm them. She could have called in and asked for sick leave or traded shifts with a co-worker—this way, the patients would not be compromised by her impaired condition. Better yet, she could have

put her job priorities ahead of her decision to go out drinking late into the evening. She could lose her job if this type of behavior happens again.

What Would You Do?

Sheila, a pharmacy technician, dropped a few capsules on the pharmacy floor while dispensing medications. Nobody else saw this happen. Quickly, she picked the capsules off the floor and put them back onto the tray, after which she included them in the container of dispensed medication. If you were Sheila, what would you do in this situation? If you were another pharmacy worker who saw this happen, what would you do?

In this situation, the pharmacist should be notified about the capsules that were dropped on the floor. They should not be used for patients after they were spilled because of possible contaminants on the floor. If Sheila had been seen dropping the pills, the person who saw this should explain to her that the pills must be discarded and not used for patients—it would be morally wrong to use them. She should be reminded that the honesty and integrity of the pharmacy staff is of utmost importance.

What Would You Do?

Mr. Johnson, who has been coming to your pharmacy for many years, approaches you. You know that his wife died the previous year, and that he is taking medications for depression as well as cancer. When he arrives with a new prescription, he asks about the prescribed medication and comments, "I sure wouldn't want to take too much of this stuff. How much of this do you think would kill me if I wasn't careful?" Do you think Mr. Johnson may be contemplating suicide? What should you do first in this situation?

Given his state of health, the death of his wife, and his depression medication, suicide may be a real concern because of his statements. As the pharmacy technician in this scenario, you should immediately notify your supervisor and/ or the pharmacist.

Chapter 3

You Be the Judge

A pharmacy technician is working on a Saturday morning. His pharmacist decides to take a break since there are no customers in the pharmacy. During the pharmacist's break, a friend of the pharmacy technician enters the pharmacy and asks if he can have a few Percocet tablets because of back pain. The pharmacy technician gives his friend six Percocet tablets out of a container in the pharmacy. His friend takes these tablets and leaves. What do you think the pharmacy technician did wrong in this situation? If the pharmacist finds out about this, what do you think the consequences will be? What possible legal action could ensue against this pharmacy technician?

The pharmacy technician has no authority to give medications to any person without a prescription. If the pharmacist finds out, the pharmacy technician will probably be fired. The pharmacist could even report the pharmacy technician to the authorities. The pharmacy technician could be charged with a

felony diversion of a controlled substance, and could be prosecuted for illegally dispensing a prescription drug. A conviction such as this would bar the pharmacy technician from participating in Medicare or Medicaid—which, in reality, means that no pharmacy would hire him in the future.

What Would You Do?

David is a pharmacy technician who received a prescription of Valium 50 mg b.i.d. for 30 days, with 5 refills. After thoroughly reviewing this prescription, if you were David, what would you do?

In this situation, the pharmacy technician should recognize that this prescription is out of the ordinary because Valium tablets are available in 2 mg, 5 mg, and 10 mg sizes, but not in 50 mg. David might assume that the physician meant to write "5.0 mg" but left out the decimal point. Also, the maximum amount of Valium usually suggested for a 1-day period is 40 mg. The pharmacy technician should report this prescription to the pharmacist immediately.

You Be the Judge

A pharmacy technician who is also an avid basketball player has begun using anabolic steroids, obtained illegally from the pharmacy in which he works. Slowly, his behavior begins to change as a result of these drugs, and he soon is fired from his job. What are the most common adverse effects of using anabolic steroids? Is the pharmacist liable for not noticing that these drugs were being taken? What would be the consequences of stealing anabolic steroids?

Anabolic steroids commonly cause hypertension, cardiac problems, mental depression, suicidal behavior, and psychosis. The pharmacist should have been aware of the missing steroids, and could be held accountable for not keeping adequate records of the drug supply in the pharmacy. The theft of anabolic steroids is a felony, punishable by 5 years or longer in prison.

What Would You Do?

Mary Jo, an inexperienced pharmacy technician, started working in a retail pharmacy last week. Many customers were in close proximity to the counter. While dispensing a prescription for a certain patient, she called out to her by name, asking, "Mrs. Corby, can you please give me your Medicaid card so that I can make a copy?" What would you do in this situation, and what law was violated by Mary Jo?

In this situation, the pharmacy technician should ask the patient for the Medicaid card without anyone else being able to hear. Though it is not a violation of HIPAA to publicly ask a patient for insurance documentation, it is polite to keep the patient's name and their insurance as confidential as possible.

CHAPTER 4

You Be the Judge

Glenn, a pharmacy technician who has been working for a year, was required because of new pharmacy rules to take drug-screening tests upon starting his second year at work. The new rules also required a full background check to be made. When Glenn's test results were returned, he had a positive result for cocaine in his system, and the background check revealed that he had a previous conviction for drug possession. In your judgment, what will be the result of Glenn's positive drug test and his background check?

If Glenn's positive drug test is against the rules of employment of the pharmacy, which is likely, he will probably be fired. If he had filled out information about his background before being hired initially, and never mentioned his drug conviction, this would also most likely result in him being fired. It is important to tell the truth about previous convictions whenever questioned about them in regard to employment.

What Would You Do?

Joe, a pharmacist, gave a list of 13 Schedule II drugs to Betty so that she could write them onto a DEA Form 222. Betty wrote all 13 items on the 10-line form so that Joe could then sign it. Joe told her she would have to redo the form. What should Betty have done in this situation?

Betty should know that only 10 items in total can be ordered on one DEA form 222. The other three items would have to be written on a second form.

What Would You Do?

Nicole had a back injury and was suffering from severe back pain. Her neurologist prescribed oxycodone for her. Two days later, her brother came to visit from out of state, planning to stay with Nicole for 1 week. Upon his arrival, he complained about a severe headache. Nicole gave some of the oxycodone to her brother to relieve his pain, which he then crushed up and snorted, similar to cocaine. Several days later, she found that five more oxycodone tablets were missing from her bottle. If you were Nicole, what would you do in this situation? Did she break the law?

Nicole should not have given the oxycodone, which is a scheduled drug, to anybody else. Distribution of this type of drug is against the law, punishable by fines and imprisonment. Though the circumstances in this situation are difficult, Nicole did break the law by giving her brother this medication.

What Would You Do?

Teresa, a pharmacy technician, was doing an initial inventory of scheduled drugs for a new pharmacy, including Schedule II drugs. She estimated the content of the scheduled drugs and recorded her estimates. When the pharmacy checked her inventory records later, he noticed that the inventory for the Schedule II drugs was not accurate. If you were Teresa, what would you have done differently?

Schedule II drugs must be counted exactly, not estimated, one by one. Schedule III, IV, and V substances may be estimated, except that Schedule III and IV bottles of 1,000 pills (or more) must be counted exactly. Teresa should have known that the Schedule II drugs required an exact count.

You Be the Judge

Monica, a pharmacy technician, has assisted the pharmacist in completing an inventory of her pharmacy's medications. She found out that one bottle containing 20 Percocet tablets was missing. She notified the pharmacist, who told her to fill out the correct DEA form, which he would then sign. Which DEA form should Monica use? What would be the next step that Monica should take?

Form 106 is the DEA form used for reporting theft or lost drugs. After filling out Form 106, the DEA and (in most areas) the local police department must be notified.

CHAPTER 5

You Be the Judge

Mr. Pelosi was admitted to Parrish Medical Center for the treatment of a sexually transmitted disease. A pharmacy technician who had access to his chart did not comply with the HIPAA Privacy Rule, and joked with a hospital janitor about Mr. Pelosi's condition. Later, the janitor, working in Mr. Pelosi's hospital room, told Mr. Pelosi not to worry, because he himself had had the same condition at one time, and that the hospital would take good care of him. Mr. Pelosi asked him how he knew about his condition, and the janitor mentioned the pharmacy technician who told him. Infuriated at this breach of his privacy, Mr. Pelosi called his lawyer and told him to file a lawsuit against the technician. In your judgment, can Mr. Pelosi sue the technician?

The HIPAA Privacy Rule does not give patients the express right to sue. The patient can file a written complaint with the Secretary of Health and Human Services through the Office of Civil Rights. The HHS Secretary then decides whether to investigate the complaint.

CHAPTER 6

What Would You Do?

While John was compounding in the laboratory, he was splashed in the eyes with a chemical. He went to the men's room and washed his face in the sink. He did not use the eyewash facilities. After going back to work, he found that his eyes remained irritated, and he could not see very well. If you were John, what would you do in this situation?

OSHA requires that eyewash facilities be available in laboratories. John should have used the eyewash facilities and notified his employer of the accident. He should have gone to the emergency room because he was still unable to see very well. His eyes could have permanent damage as a result.

What Would You Do?

Mary, a pharmacy technician working in a hospital pharmacy, was splashed when she accidentally dropped a glass medication bottle into an airflow hood. The moving air carried the medication onto her face. She was not wearing a mask but was wearing protective glasses. The medication partially entered into her nose. If you were Mary, what would you do in this situation?

After exposure, Mary should immediately follow the post-exposure procedures of her hospital pharmacy, and notify her supervisor.

You Be the Judge

A compounding pharmacy provided its workers with gowns, goggles, gloves, and similar equipment on a regular basis, but did not provide an airflow hood because the types of substances compounded there did not require such a device. Because of a fire that occurred in a nearby compounding pharmacy, this pharmacy was asked to quickly handle the compounding for cytotoxic agents required for several different patients. A pharmacy technician who knew that an airflow hood was required for these agents refused to complete the compounding, and was reprimanded. He notified OSHA that the pharmacist was completing the compounding of cytotoxic agents without the proper equipment. What do you think the OSHA inspectors would do in this case?

In this case, OSHA would hold the pharmacist accountable for the illegal compounding of cytotoxic agents without the proper equipment. The pharmacy technician was correct in his assumption about OSHA rules. Most likely, the pharmacist would be fined for his actions.

What Would You Do?

Shannon was working with electronic equipment in her pharmacy when a power cord caught fire. She was extremely nervous, and could not remember what she should do in case of fire. If you were Shannon, what procedures do you think she should follow?

Shannon should pull the fire alarm box to alert her fellow employees of the fire. She should then locate the closest fire extinguisher by using the fire safety plan (which should show fire extinguisher locations).

What Would You Do?

Mark is a pharmacy technician. Three weeks after he was hired, his pharmacist set up an OSHA training class. Mark was sick during this time, and unable to attend. On his first day back at work, he was attempting to clean up a corrosive chemical spill on the floor. Since he had missed the training, Mark was unsure of the proper procedures to follow, and wore latex gloves while cleaning up the spill. If you were Mark, what would you do in this situation?

If Mark had attended his OSHA training, he would have known that special thick gloves are required to be used when cleaning up corrosive chemical spills, not ordinary latex gloves, which these types of chemicals can burn through. Therefore, only special utility gloves that resist corrosive chemicals should be used. If Mark was injured as a result, the pharmacy would be responsible. They should not have allowed Mark, who did not receive the training, to clean up the spill.

You Be the Judge

Joshua took a special OSHA course and understood his responsibilities on the job. One day, he was doing his routine work and dealing with chemical substances. He did not use protective equipment for safety. What could be the result of Joshua's actions?

Joshua could have been exposed to biohazards. Routine activities at work do not warrant the lack of protective equipment because accidents can happen at any time. He should always wear protective equipment when dealing with chemical substances, no matter how routine the work may be.

What Would You Do?

Richard was talking to one of his co-workers, Nicole, in the pharmacy. He told her a rather rude joke of a sexual nature. Nicole was offended by the joke. If you were Nicole, what would you do?

Nicole has several options in this situation. She could ask Richard not to tell her any more jokes of this nature. If Richard persisted with these kinds of jokes, Nicole could report his actions to her supervisor, and even the authorities.

CHAPTER 7

What Would You Do?

Tara is a pharmacy technician who recently moved from Maine to Florida. According to the National Association of Boards of Pharmacy, if you were Tara, what must you do in order to be able to practice in Florida?

In this situation, a pharmacy technician can simply apply for any open position. The State of Florida previously did not require certification or registration in order to be able to practice as a pharmacy technician. (However, as of July 2008, Florida is now requiring PTCB certification for pharmacy technicians.) If Tara already had previous certification or registration in another state, her qualifications may help her to gain employment more quickly than other applicants who may be uncertified or unregistered. Tara must get information about her Boards of Pharmacy, registration, continuing education, disciplinary actions, and status of pharmacy technicians.

You Be the Judge

A new drug store was about to open in Minnesota. The pharmacist tried to follow the minimum requirements of his state. The store opened and, soon after, was inspected by the State Board of Pharmacy. The inspector discovered that the fire safety and hazard communication plans were not in place. What would be the consequences of this situation?

The State Board of Pharmacy may not allow the pharmacy to open until a correct fire safety plan and hazard communication is established, and the proper displays are posted. This includes evacuation routes, fire alarm pull states, locations of extinguishers, etc.

What Would You Do?

Tina, a pharmacy technician, was dispensing a sulfa drug prescription. She forgot to put a required auxiliary label onto the container. The pharmacist noticed that there was no auxiliary label and told Tina that she must put the appropriate label onto the container. If you were Tina, what should you know about sulfa drugs and related auxiliary labels?

Sulfa drugs can cause severe adverse effects on the kidneys. The auxiliary label should indicate that this drug must be taken with plenty of water. Also, direct sunlight should be avoided as much as possible when taking sulfa drugs, and appropriate labeling regarding this point should be included.

You Be the Judge

Your pharmacist received a prescription for Zocor® 20 mg for 30 days. He selected the generic drug, simvastatin, instead of Zocor. Based on your knowledge, why did the pharmacist make this substitution? Is he allowed to do this?

The pharmacist followed a generic substitution law allowing simvastatin to be substituted for Zocor (if authorized by the physician) in order to save the patient money. Simvastatin is identical to Zocor, so the pharmacist is allowed to make this substitution.

What Would You Do?

While you are dispensing a drug product, you hear that a client has asked the pharmacist if he can purchase a dozen hypodermic needles and syringes. The client claims he is a diabetic. You know this client personally, and are sure of his illegal drug use in the past. What would you do in this scenario?

Morally, you are obligated to alert the pharmacist about the client's request, because sometimes the pharmacist requires a prescription for needles and syringes. However, since some states do not require a prescription for obtaining hypodermic or insulin needles and syringes, this patient may be able to obtain them regardless. Certain state law holds that these devices need to be available for sale without prescription because patients such as diabetics may need them quickly. A diabetic individual would probably know that he should ask for "insulin" syringes and not "hypodermic" syringes.

CHAPTER 8

What Would You Do?

Sean has been working in a retail pharmacy for 10 years. His certification has expired and he must renew it quickly in order to continue to practice.

If you were Sean, what must you do to renew your certification?

Renewal of certification requires that the applicant complete 20 hours of continuing education credits every 2 years (1 hour of which must focus on pharmacy law), updating of the applicant's information with the certifying agency, paying a renewal fee, and filling out a renewal application form, which must be submitted per individual state time requirements. If late, the renewal may also require an additional fee. Also, it is important to remember that Sean cannot legally practice while his certification is expired.

You Be the Judge

Betty, a pharmacy technician, is working in a hospital pharmacy. While she is repacking drugs, she discovers that some of them have defective packaging. However, she ignores this, and repacks the drugs anyway. What do you think that Betty should have done in this case?

Betty should have notified her pharmacist about the defective packaging. Then, the decision could have been made to return them to the manufacturer or distributor in exchange for properly packaged replacements. If the defective packaging has damaged the drugs in any way, their effectiveness could be compromised, resulting in a medication error. Knowledge of the defective packaging and Betty's actions could result in penalties being assessed against Betty, the pharmacist, and the pharmacy itself.

Medication Errors (MedWatch)

MedWatch is the FDA's Medical Products Reporting Program. It is a voluntary system that healthcare providers can use to report problems to the FDA. Also, manufacturers and distributors of FDA-approved biologics, drugs, special nutritional products, dietary supplements, radiation-emitting devices, infant formulas, and other devices must report related problems and errors to the FDA. The form that is used to report problems and errors is shown below. (Source: http://www.fda.gov/medwatch.)

ADVICE ABOUT VOLUNTARY REPORTING

Detailed instructions available at: http://www.fda.gov/medwatch/report/consumer/instruct.htm

Report adverse events, product problems or product use errors with:

- Medications *(drugs or biologics)*
- Medical devices *(including in-vitro diagnostics)*
- Combination products *(medication & medical devices)*
- Human cells, tissues, and cellular and tissue-based products
- Special nutritional products *(dietary supplements, medical foods, infant formulas)*
- Cosmetics

Report product problems - quality, performance or safety concerns such as:

- Suspected counterfeit product
- Suspected contamination
- Questionable stability
- Defective components
- Poor packaging or labeling
- Therapeutic failures (product didn't work)

Report SERIOUS adverse events. An event is serious when the patient outcome is:

- Death
- Life-threatening
- Hospitalization - initial or prolonged
- Disability or permanent damage
- Congenital anomaly/birth defect
- Required intervention to prevent permanent impairment or damage
- Other serious (important medical events)

Report even if:

- You're not certain the product caused the event
- You don't have all the details

How to report:

- Just fill in the sections that apply to your report
- Use section D for all products except medical devices
- Attach additional pages if needed
- Use a separate form for each patient
- Report either to FDA or the manufacturer *(or both)*

Other methods of reporting:

- 1-800-FDA-0178 -- To FAX report
- 1-800-FDA-1088 -- To report by phone
- www.fda.gov/medwatch/report.htm -- To report online

If your report involves a serious adverse event with a device and it occurred in a facility outside a doctor's office, that facility may be legally required to report to FDA and/or the manufacturer. Please notify the person in that facility who would handle such reporting.

If your report involves a serious adverse event with a vaccine call 1-800-822-7967 to report.

Confidentiality: The patient's identity is held in strict confidence by FDA and protected to the fullest extent of the law. FDA will not disclose the reporter's identity in response to a request from the public, pursuant to the Freedom of Information Act. The reporter's identity, including the identity of a self-reporter, may be shared with the manufacturer unless requested otherwise.

The public reporting burden for this collection of information has been estimated to average 36 minutes per response, including the time for reviewing instructions, searching existing data sources, gathering and maintaining the data needed, and completing and reviewing the collection of information. Send comments regarding this burden estimate or any other aspect of this collection of information, including suggestions for reducing this burden to:

Department of Health and Human Services	*Please DO NOT*	*OMB statement:*
Food and Drug Administration - MedWatch	*RETURN this form*	*"An agency may not conduct or sponsor, and a*
10903 New Hampshire Avenue	*to this address.*	*person is not required to respond to, a collection of*
Building 22, Mail Stop 4447		*information unless it displays a currently valid*
Silver Spring, MD 20993-0002		*OMB control number."*

U.S. DEPARTMENT OF HEALTH AND HUMAN SERVICES
Food and Drug Administration

FORM FDA 3500 (10/05) (Back)   Please Use Address Provided Below -- Fold in Thirds, Tape and Mail

---

**DEPARTMENT OF
HEALTH & HUMAN SERVICES**

Public Health Service
Food and Drug Administration
Rockville, MD 20857

Official Business
Penalty for Private Use $300

NO POSTAGE
NECESSARY
IF MAILED
IN THE
UNITED STATES
OR APO/FPO

BUSINESS REPLY MAIL
FIRST CLASS MAIL   PERMIT NO. 946   ROCKVILLE MD

MEDWATCH
The FDA Safety Information and Adverse Event Reporting Program
Food and Drug Administration
5600 Fishers Lane
Rockville, MD 20852-9787

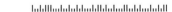

Special Tasks for Pharmacy Technicians in Community Settings

State	May Prepare Medications in Cards for Nursing Homes	May Reconstitute Oral Liquids	May Place Prescription Labels on Containers	May Call Physicians for Refill Authorization
Alabama	Yes	Yes	Yes	Yes
Alaska	Yes	Yes	Yes	Yes
Arizona	Yes	Yes	Yes	Yes
Arkansas	Yes	Yes	Yes	Yes
California	Yes	Yes	Yes	Yes
Colorado	Yes	Yes	Yes	Yes
Connecticut	Yes	Yes	Yes	Yes
Delaware	Yes	Yes	Yes	No
District of Columbia	Yes	Yes	Yes	Yes
Florida	Yes	Yes	Yes	Yes
Georgia	Yes	Yes	Yes	No
Hawaii	Yes	Yes	Yes	No
Idaho	Yes	Yes	Yes	Yes
Illinois	Yes	Yes	Yes	Yes
Indiana	Yes	Yes	Yes	Yes
Iowa	Yes	Yes	Yes	Yes
Kansas	Yes	Yes	Yes	Yes
Kentucky	Yes	Yes	Yes	Yes
Louisiana	Yes	Yes	Yes	Yes
Maine	Yes	Yes	Yes	Yes
Maryland	Yes	Yes	Yes	No
Massachusetts	Yes	Yes	Yes	Yes
Michigan	Yes	Yes	Yes	No
Minnesota	Yes	Yes	Yes	Yes
Mississippi	Yes	Yes	Yes	Yes
Missouri	Yes	Yes	Yes	Yes

(continued)

State	May Prepare Medications in Cards for Nursing Homes	May Reconstitute Oral Liquids	May Place Prescription Labels on Containers	May Call Physicians for Refill Authorization
Montana	Yes	Yes	Yes	No
Nebraska	Yes	Yes	Yes	No
Nevada	Yes	Yes	Yes	Yes
New Hampshire	Yes	Yes	Yes	No
New Jersey	Yes	Yes	Yes	No
New Mexico	Yes	Yes	Yes	Yes
New York	Yes	No	Yes	No
North Carolina	Yes	Yes	Yes	Yes
North Dakota	Yes	Yes	Yes	Yes
Ohio	Yes	Yes	Yes	No
Oklahoma	Yes	Yes	Yes	Yes
Oregon	Yes	Yes	Yes	Yes
Pennsylvania	Yes	Yes	Yes	No
Rhode Island	Yes	Yes	Yes	Yes
South Carolina	Yes	Yes	Yes	No
South Dakota	Yes	Yes	Yes	No
Tennessee	Yes	Yes	Yes	Yes
Texas	Yes	Yes	Yes	Yes
Utah	Yes	Yes	Yes	Yes
Vermont	Yes	Yes	Yes	Yes
Virginia	Yes	Yes	Yes	No
Washington	Yes	Yes	Yes	Yes
West Virginia	Yes	Yes	Yes	Yes
Wisconsin	Yes	No	Yes	Yes
Wyoming	Yes	Yes	Yes	Yes

Source: *Adapted from Strandberg, K. M. (2002). Essentials of Law and Ethics for Pharmacy Technicians. New York: CRC Press.*

State-by-State Approved Duties of Pharmacy Technicians in Hospital Settings

State	Accept Phoned Prescriptions	Enter Prescriptions into Computer	Enter Information into Patient Files	Retrieve Stocked Medications	Prepare Prescription Labels	Place Medications into Containers
Alabama	No	Yes	Yes	Yes	Yes	Yes
Alaska	No	Yes	Yes	Yes	Yes	Yes
Arizona	No	Yes	Yes	Yes	Yes	Yes
Arkansas	No	Yes	Yes	Yes	Yes	Yes
California	No	Yes	Yes	Yes	Yes	Yes
Colorado	No	Yes	Yes	Yes	Yes	Yes
Connecticut	No	Yes	Yes	Yes	Yes	Yes
Delaware	No	Yes	Yes	Yes	Yes	Yes
District of Columbia	Yes	Yes	Yes	Yes	Yes	Yes
Florida	No	Yes	Yes	Yes	Yes	Yes
Georgia	No	Yes	Yes	Yes	Yes	Yes
Hawaii	No	Yes	Yes	Yes	Yes	Yes
Idaho	No	Yes	Yes	Yes	Yes	Yes
Illinois	No	Yes	Yes	Yes	Yes	Yes
Indiana	No	Yes	Yes	Yes	Yes	Yes
Iowa	Yes	Yes	Yes	Yes	Yes	Yes
Kansas	No	Yes	Yes	Yes	Yes	Yes
Kentucky	No	Yes	Yes	Yes	Yes	Yes
Louisiana	No	Yes	Yes	Yes	Yes	Yes
Maine	No	Yes	Yes	Yes	Yes	Yes
Maryland	No	Yes	Yes	Yes	Yes	Yes
Massachusetts	No	Yes	Yes	Yes	Yes	Yes
Michigan	Yes	Yes	Yes	Yes	Yes	Yes
Minnesota	No	Yes	Yes	Yes	Yes	Yes
Mississippi	No	Yes	Yes	Yes	Yes	Yes
Missouri	Yes	Yes	Yes	Yes	Yes	Yes
Montana	No	Yes	Yes	Yes	Yes	Yes

(continued)

State	Accept Phoned Prescriptions	Enter Prescriptions into Computer	Enter Information into Patient Files	Retrieve Stocked Medications	Prepare Prescription Labels	Place Medications into Containers
Nebraska	No	Yes	Yes	Yes	Yes	Yes
Nevada	No	Yes	Yes	Yes	Yes	Yes
New Hampshire	No	Yes	Yes	Yes	Yes	Yes
New Jersey	No	Yes	Yes	Yes	Yes	Yes
New Mexico	No	Yes	Yes	Yes	Yes	Yes
New York	No	Yes	Yes	Yes	Yes	Yes
North Carolina	Yes	Yes	Yes	Yes	Yes	Yes
North Dakota	Yes	Yes	Yes	Yes	Yes	Yes
Ohio	No	Yes	Yes	Yes	Yes	Yes
Oklahoma	No	Yes	Yes	Yes	Yes	Yes
Oregon	No	Yes	Yes	Yes	Yes	Yes
Pennsylvania	No	Yes	Yes	Yes	Yes	Yes
Rhode Island	Yes	Yes	Yes	Yes	Yes	Yes
South Carolina	No	Yes	Yes	Yes	Yes	Yes
South Dakota	No	No	Yes	Yes	Yes	Yes
Tennessee	Yes	Yes	Yes	Yes	Yes	Yes
Texas	No	Yes	Yes	Yes	Yes	Yes
Utah	No	Yes	Yes	Yes	Yes	Yes
Vermont	No	Yes	Yes	Yes	Yes	Yes
Virginia	No	Yes	Yes	Yes	Yes	Yes
Washington	No	Yes	Yes	Yes	Yes	Yes
West Virginia	No	Yes	Yes	Yes	Yes	Yes
Wisconsin	No	Yes	Yes	Yes	Yes	Yes
Wyoming	No	Yes	Yes	Yes	Yes	Yes

Source: *Adapted from Strandberg, K. M. (2002). Essentials of Law and Ethics for Pharmacy Technicians. New York: CRC Press.*

State Qualifications for Pharmacy Technicians

State	State Certified?	State Registered?	State Licensed?
Alabama	No	Yes	No
Alaska	No	No	Yes
Arizona	No	No	Yes
Arkansas	No	Yes	No
California	No	Yes	Yes
Colorado	No	No	No
Connecticut	No	Yes	No
Delaware	No	No	No
District of Columbia	Yes, as of 2008	No	No
Florida	Yes, as of 2008	Yes, as of 2010	No
Georgia	No	No	No
Hawaii	No	No	No
Idaho	No	Yes	No
Illinois	No	Yes	No
Indiana	Yes	No	No
Iowa	No, will change in 2010	Yes	No
Kansas	No	Yes	No
Kentucky	No, but currently in negotiation	No, but currently in negotiation	No, but currently in negotiation
Louisiana	Yes	No	No
Maine	No	Yes	No
Maryland	No	Yes	No
Massachusetts	No	Yes	No
Michigan	No	No	No
Minnesota	No	Yes	No
Mississippi	No	Yes	No

(continued)

State	State Certified?	State Registered?	State Licensed?
Missouri	No	Yes	No
Montana	Yes	Yes	No
Nebraska	No	No	No
Nevada	No	Yes	No
New Hampshire	No	Yes	No
New Jersey	No	Yes	No
New Mexico	No	Yes	No
New York	No	No	No
North Carolina	No	Yes	No
North Dakota	No	Yes	No
Ohio	No	No	No
Oklahoma	No	Yes	No
Oregon	No	No	Yes
Pennsylvania	No	No	No
Rhode Island	No	Yes	Yes
South Carolina	Yes	Yes	No
South Dakota	No	Yes	No
Tennessee	No	Yes	No
Texas	No	Yes	No
Utah	No	No	Yes
Vermont	No	Yes	No
Virginia	No	Yes	No
Washington	Yes	No	No
West Virginia	No	Yes	No
Wisconsin	No	No	No
Wyoming	No	Yes	Yes

Source: *Adapted from Strandberg, K. M. (2002). Essentials of Law and Ethics for Pharmacy Technicians. New York: CRC Press.*

State Boards of Pharmacy

National Association of Boards of Pharmacy
Carmen A. Catizone, Executive Director/Secretary
1600 Feehanville Drive
Mount Prospect, IL 60056
Phone: 847/391-4406
Web site: http://www.nabp.net
E-mail: exec-office@nabp.net

Alabama
Herbert "Herb" Bobo, Executive Director
10 Inverness Center, Suite 110
Birmingham, AL 35242
Phone: 205/981-2280
Web site: http://www.albop.com
E-mail: hbobo@albop.com

Alaska
Sher Zinn, Licensing Examiner
PO Box 110806
Juneau, AK 99811-0806
Phone: 907/465-2589
Web site: http://www.commerce.state.ak.us/
   occ/ppha.htm
E-mail: sher.zinn@alaska.gov

Arizona
Hal Wand, Executive Director
1700 W Washington St., Suite 250
Phoenix, AZ 85007
Phone: 602/771-2727
Web site: http://www.azpharmacy.gov
E-mail: chunter@azpharmacy.gov

Arkansas
Charles S. Campbell, Executive Director
101 E Capitol, Suite 218
Little Rock, AR 72201
Phone: 501/682-0190
Web site: http://www.arkansas.gov/asbp
E-mail: Charlie.Campbell@arkansas.gov

California
Virginia "Giny" Herold, Executive Officer
1625 N Market Blvd., Suite N219
Sacramento, CA 95834
Phone: 916/574-7912
Web site: http://www.pharmacy.ca.gov
E-mail: Virginia_herold@dca.ca.gov

Colorado
Wendy Anderson, Program Director
1560 Broadway, Suite 1300
Denver, CO 80202-5143
Phone: 303/894-7800
Web site: http://www.dora.state.co.us/pharmacy/
E-mail: pharmacy@dora.state.co.us

Connecticut
Delinda Brown-Jagne, Board Administrator
165 Capital Avenue, Room 147
Hartford, CT 06106
Phone: 860/713-6070
Web site: http://www.ct.gov/dcp/site/default.asp
E-mail: delina.brown-jagne@ct.gov

Delaware
David W. Dryden, Executive Secretary
861 Silver Lake Blvd., Suite 203
Dover, DE 19904
Phone: 302/744-4526
Web site: http://dpr.delaware.gov/boards/pharmacy/
   newpharmacy.shtml
E-mail: debop@state.de.us

District of Columbia
Marcia B. Wooden, Executive Director
717 – 14th St NW, Suite 600
Washington, D.C. 20005
Phone: 202/442-4762
Web site: http://hpla.doh.dc.gov/hpla/cwp/
E-mail: Marcia.wooden@dc.gov

Florida
Rebecca Poston, Executive Director
4052 Bald Cypress Way, Bin #C04
Tallahassee, FL 32399-3254
Phone: 850/245-4292
Web site: http://www.doh.state.fl.us/mqa/pharmacy/
E-mail: MQA_Pharmacy@doh.state.fl.us

Georgia
Lisa Durden, Executive Director
237 Coliseum Dr
Macon, GA 31217-3858
Phone: 478/207-2440
Web site: http://www.sos.ga.gov/plb/pharmacy/
E-mail: http://sos.georgia.gov/cgi-bin/email.asp

Guam
Jane M. Diego, Secretary for the Board
PO Box 2816
Hagatna, GU 96932
Phone: 671/735-7406 ext 11
Web site: http://www.dphss.guam.gov/
E-mail: jane.diego@dphss.guam.gov

Hawaii
Lee Ann Teshima, Executive Officer
PO Box 3469
Honolulu, HI 96801
Phone: 808/586-2694
Web site: http://www.hawaii.gov/dcca/areas/pvl/
   boards/pharmacy
E-mail: pharmacy@dcca.hawaii.gov

Idaho
Mark D. Johnston, Executive Director
3380 Americana Terrace, Suite 320
Boise, ID 83706
Phone: 208/334-2356
Web site: http://www.accessidaho.org/bop/
E-mail: info@bop.idaho.gov

Illinois
Kim Scott, Pharmacy Board Liaison
320 W Washington, 3rd Floor
Springfield, IL 62786
Phone: 217/782-8556
Web site: http://www.idfpr.com
E-mail: fpr.prfgroup10@illinois.gov

Indiana
Marty Allain, Director
402 W Washington St, Room W072
Indianapolis, IN 46204-2739
Phone: 317/234-2067
Web site: http://www.in.gov/pla/2361.htm
E-mail: pla4@pla.IN.gov

Iowa
Lloyd K. Jessen, Executive Director/Secretary
400 SW 8th St, Suite E
Des Moines, IA 50309-4688
Phone: 515/281-5944
Web site: http://www.state.ia.us/ibpe
E-mail: lloyd.jessen@iowa.gov

Kansas
Debra L. Billingsley, Executive Secretary
Landon State Office Building, 900 SW Jackson, Room
    560
Topeka, KS 66612-1231
Phone: 785/296-4056
Web site: http://www.kansas.gov/pharmacy
E-mail: dbillingsley@pharmacy.ks.gov

Kentucky
Michael A. Burleson, Executive Director
Spindletop Administration Bldg, Suite 302,
2624 Research Park Dr,
Lexington, KY 40511
Phone: 859/246-2820
Web site: http://pharmacy.ky.gov/
E-mail: pharmacy.board@ky.gov

Louisiana
Malcolm J. Broussard, Executive Director
5615 Corporate Blvd, Suite 8E
Baton Rouge, LA 70808-2537
Phone: 225/925-6496
Web site: http://www.labp.com
E-mail: exec@labp.com

Maine
Geraldine L."Jeri" Betts, Board Administrator
35 State House Station
Augusta, ME 04333
Phone: 207/624-8603
Web site: http://www.maine.gov/professionallicensing
E-mail: geraldine.l.betts@maine.gov

Maryland
La Verne George Naesea, Executive Director
4201 Patterson Ave
Baltimore, MD 21215-2299
Phone: 410/764-4755
Web site: http://www.dhmh.state.md.us/
    pharmacyboard/
E-mail: mdbop@dhmh.state.md.us

Massachusetts
James D. Coffey, Director
239 Causeway St, 2nd Floor, Suite 200
Boston, MA 02114
Phone: 617/973-0950
Web site: http://www.mass.gov/reg/boards/ph
E-mail: James.d.coffey@state.ma.us

Michigan
Rae Ramsdell, Director, Licensing Division
611 W Ottawa, First Floor
PO Box 30670
Lansing, MI 48909-8170
Phone: 517/335-0918
Web site: http://www.michigan.gov/
    healthlicense
E-mail: rhramsd@michigan.gov

Minnesota
Cody C. Wiberg, Executive Director
2829 University Ave SE, Suite 530
Minneapolis, MN 55414-3251
Phone: 651/201-2825
Web site: http://www.phcybrd.state.mn.us
E-mail: pharmacy.board@state.mn.us

Mississippi
Leland "Mac" McDivitt, Executive Director
204 Key Dr, Suite D
Madison, MS 39110
Phone: 601/605-5388
Web site: http://www.mbp.state.ms.us
E-mail: lmcdivitt@mbp.state.ms.us

Missouri
Debra C. Ringgenberg, Executive Director
PO Box 625
Jefferson City, MO 65102
Phone: 573/751-0091
Web site: http://www.pr.mo.gov/pharmacists.asp
E-mail: pharmacy@pr.mo.gov

Montana
Ronald J. Klein, Executive Director
PO Box 200513
301 S Park Ave, 4th Floor
Helena, MT 59620-0513
Phone: 406/841-2371
Web site: http://mt.gov/dli/bsd/license/bsd_boards/
    pha_board/board_page.asp
E-mail: roklein@mt.gov

Nebraska
Becky Wisell, Administrator
PO Box 94986
Lincoln, NE 68509-4986
Phone: 402/471-2118
Web site: http://www.hhs.state.ne.us
E-mail: becky.wisell@dhhs.ne.gov

Nevada
Larry L. Pinson, Executive Secretary
431 W Plumb Lane
Reno, NV 89509
Phone: 775/850-1440
Web site: http://bop.nv.gov
E-mail: pharmacy@pharmacy.nv.gov

New Hampshire
Paul G. Boisseau, Executive Secretary
57 Regional Dr
Concord, NH 03301-8518
Phone: 603/271-2350
Web site: http://www.nh.gov/pharmacy
E-mail: pharmacy.board@nh.gov

New Jersey
Joanne Boyer, Executive Director
PO Box 45013
Newark, NJ 07101
Phone: 973/504-6450
Web site: http://www.state.nj.us/lps/ca/boards.htm
E-mail: boyerj@dca.lps.state.nj.us

New Mexico
William Harvey, Executive Director/Chief
    Drug Inspector
5200 Oakland NE, Suite A
Albuquerque, NM 87113
Phone: 505/222-9830
Web site: http://www.rld.state.nm.us/Pharmacy/
E-mail: pharmacy.board@state.nm.us

New York
Lawrence H. Mokhiber, Executive Secretary
89 Washington Ave, 2nd Floor W
Albany, NY 12234-1000
Phone: 518/474-3817 ext. 130
Web site: www.op.nysed.gov
E-mail: pharmbd@mail.nysed.gov

North Carolina
Jack W. "Jay" Campbell IV, Executive Director
PO Box 4560
Chapel Hill, NC 27515-4560
Phone: 919/246-1050
Web site: http://www.ncbop.org
E-mail: jcampbell@ncbop.org

North Dakota
Howard C. Anderson, Jr., Executive Director
1906 E Broadway Ave
Bismarck, ND 58501-1354
Phone: 701/328-9535
Web site: http://www.nodakpharmacy.com
E-mail: ndboph@btinet.net

Ohio
William T. Winsley, Executive Director
77 S High St, Room 1702
Columbus, OH 43215-6126
Phone: 614/466-4143
Web site: http://www.pharmacy.ohio.gov
E-mail: exec@bop.state.oh.us

Oklahoma
Bryan H. Potter, Executive Director
4545 Lincoln Blvd, Suite 112
Oklahoma City, OK 73105-3488
Phone: 405/521-3815
Web site: http://www.pharmacy.ok.gov
E-mail: pharmacy@pharmacy.ok.gov

Oregon
Gary A. Schnabel, Executive Director
800 NE Oregon St, Suite 150
Portland, OR 97232
Phone: 971/673-0001
Web site: http://www.pharmacy.state.or.us
E-mail: pharmacy.board@state.or.us

Pennsylvania
Melanie Zimmerman, Executive Secretary
PO Box 2649
Harrisburg, PA 17105-2649
Phone: 717/783-7156
Web site: http://www.dos.state.pa.us/pharm
E-mail: st-pharmacy@state.pa.us

Puerto Rico
Magda Bouet, Executive Director,
    Department of Health
Call Box 10200
Santurce, PR 00908
Phone: 787/725-7506
Web site: http://www.salud.gov/pr/Pages/default.
    aspx
E-mail: mbouet@salud.gov.pr

Rhode Island
Catherine A. Cordy, Executive Director
3 Capitol Hill, Room 205
Providence, RI 02908-5097
Phone: 401/222-2840
Web site: http://www.health.ri.gov/hsr/professions/
    pharmacy.php
E-mail: cathyc@doh.state.ri.us

South Carolina
Lee Ann Bundrick, Administrator
110 Centerview Dr, Suite 306
Columbia, SC 29210
Phone: 803/896-4700
Web site: http://www.llronline.com/POL/pharmacy
E-mail: bundricl@llr.sc.gov

South Dakota
Ronald J. Huether, Executive Secretary
4305 S Louise Ave, Suite 104
Sioux Falls, SD 57106
Phone: 605/362-2737
Web site: http://www.pharmacy.sd.gov
E-mail: ronald.huether@state.sd.us

Tennessee
Kevin K. Eidson, Executive Director
227 French Landing, Suite 300
Nashville, TN 37243
Phone: 615/741-2718
Web site: http://health.state.tn.us/Boards/Pharmacy/
    index.shtml
E-mail: kevin.eidson@state.tn.us

Texas
Gay Dodson, Executive Director/Secretary
333 Guadalupe, Tower 3, Suite 600
Austin, TX 78701-3943
Phone: 512/305-8000
Web site: http://www.tsbp.state.tx.us
E-mail: gay.dodson@tsbp.state.tx.us

Utah
Noel Taxin, Bureau Manager
PO Box 146741
Salt Lake City, UT 84114-6741
Phone: 801/530-6621
Web site: http://www.dopl.utah.gov/
E-mail: ntaxin@utah.gov

Vermont
Peggy Atkins, Board Administrator
National Life Bldg, North FL2
Montpelier, VT 05620-3402
Phone: 802/828-2373
Web site: http://www.vtprofessionals.org
E-mail: patkins@sec.state.vt.us

Virgin Islands
Lydia T. Scott, Executive Assistant
48 Sugar Estate
St. Thomas, VI 00802
Phone: 340/774-0117
Web site: http://www.healthvi.org
E-mail: lydia.scott@usvi-doh.org

Virginia
Elizabeth Scott Russell, Executive Director
9960 Mayland Drive, Suite 300
Richmond, VA 23233-1463
Phone: 804/367-4456
Web site: http://www.dhp.virginia.gov/pharmacy
E-mail: pharmbd@dhp.virginia.gov

Washington
Steven M. Saxe, Executive Director
PO Box 47863
Olympia, WA 98504-7863
Phone: 360/236-4825
Web site: https://fortress.wa.gov/doh/hpqa1/hps4/
    pharmacy/default.htm
E-mail: steven.saxe@doh.wa.gov

West Virginia
David E. Potters, Executive Director and General
    Counsel
232 Capitol St
Charleston, WV 25301
Phone: 304/558-0558
Web site: http://www.wvbop.com/
E-mail: dpotters@wvbop.com

Wisconsin
Thomas Ryan, Bureau Director
PO Box 8935
Madison, WI 53708-8935
Phone: 608/266-2112
Web site: http://www.drl.state.wi.us/
E-mail: thomas.ryan@drl.state.wi.us

Wyoming
Mary K. Walker, Executive Director
632 S David St
Casper, WY 82601
Phone: 307/234-0294
Web site: http://pharmacyboard.state.wy.us/
E-mail: wybop@state.wy.us

Source: http://www.nabp.net

Professional Organizations

American Association of Colleges of Pharmacy (AACP)
1727 King Street
Alexandria, VA 22314
(703) 739-2330
http://www.aacp.org
Established in 1900, the AACP represents all 105 pharmacy colleges and schools in the United States.

American Association of Pharmaceutical Scientists (AAPS)
2107 Wilson Blvd., Suite 700
Arlington, VA 22201-3042
(703) 243-2800
http://www.aaps.org
Established in 1986, the AAPS provides an international forum for the exchange of knowledge among scientists to enhance their contributions to public health. The AAPS publishes the following journals: *Pharmaceutical Research*, *Pharmaceutical Development* and *Technology*, *AAPSPharmSciTech*, and *The AAPS Journal*.

American Association of Pharmacy Technicians (AAPT)
PO Box 1447
Greensboro, NC 27402
(877) 368-4771
http://www.pharmacytechnician.com
Established in 1979, the AAPT promotes the safe, efficacious, and cost-effective dispensing, distribution, and use of medicines.

American College of Clinical Pharmacy (ACCP)
13000 W 87th St Parkway
Lenexa, KS 66215-4530
(913) 492-3311

http://www.accp.com
Established in 1979, the ACCP is a professional, scientific society that provides leadership, education, advocacy, and resources that enable clinical pharmacists to achieve excellence in practice and research.

American Council on Pharmaceutical Education (ACPE)
20 North Clark Street, Suite 2500
Chicago, IL 60602-5109
(312) 664-3575
http://www.acpe-accredit.org
Also referred to as the "Accreditation Council on Pharmaceutical Education," the ACPE was established in 1932 and is the national agency for the accreditation of professional degree programs in pharmacy and of providers of continuing pharmacy education.

American Pharmacists Association (APhA)
1100 15th Street NW, Suite 400
Washington, DC 20005-1707
(202) 628-4410
http://www.aphanet.org
Established in 1852 as the American Pharmaceutical Association, the APhA is a leader in providing professional education and information for pharmacists and is an advocate for improved health of the American public through the provision of comprehensive pharmaceutical care. The APhA consists of three academies:

- The Academy of Pharmacy Practice and Management (APhA-APPM)
- The Academy of Pharmaceutical Research and Science (APhA-APRS)
- The Academy of Students of Pharmacy (APhA-APS)

American Society of Health-System Pharmacists (ASHP)

7272 Wisconsin Avenue
Bethesda, MD 20814
(301) 657-3000
http://www.ashp.org
Established in 1942, the ASHP believes that the mission of pharmacists is to help people make the best use of medications. They strive to assist pharmacists in fulfilling this mission. The ASHP represents pharmacists who practice in:

- Health maintenance organizations (HMOs)
- Hospitals
- Home care agencies
- Long-term care facilities
- Other institutions

National Pharmacy Technicians Association (NPTA)

PO Box 683148
Houston, TX 72268
(888) 247-8700
http://www.pharmacytechnician.org
Established in 1991, the NPTA serves to provide education, advocacy, and support to pharmacy technicians.

Pharmacy Technician Certification Board (PTCB)

1100 15th St NW, Suite 730
Washington, DC 20005-1707
(800) 363-8012
http://www.ptcb.org
Established in 1941, the PTCB develops, maintains, promotes, and administers a high-quality certification and recertification program for pharmacy technicians.

Pharmacy Technician Educators Council (PTEC)

6144 Knyghton Road
Indianapolis, IN 46220
(317) 962-0919
http://www.rxptec.org
Established in 1991, the PTEC strives to assist the profession of pharmacy in preparing high-quality, well-trained personnel through education and practical training.

United States Pharmacopoeia (USP)

12601 Twinbrook Parkway
Rockville, MD 20852-1790
(800) 227-8772
http://www.usp.org
Established in 1820, the USP is the official public standards-setting authority for all prescription and over-the-counter medications, dietary supplements, and other health-care products manufactured and sold in the United States.

United States Pharmacopoeia (USP) and National Formulary (NF) Drug Monograph Sample

The United States Pharmacopoeia (USP) was established to ensure the quality of medicines and health care technologies. The USP publishes the USP-NF (United States Pharmacopoeia and National Formulary). The USP-NF contains monographs that include requirements and test procedures for many food and drug substances. Monographs consist of:

- A substance's molecular structure
- A substance's chemical formula and molecular weight
- The required potency for a substance to be considered "USP grade"
- Packaging and storage requirements
- Labeling requirements
- USP reference standards required for testing a substance
- Description of test methods, references to test methods, and references to related monographs

The USP-NF also contains descriptions of analytical procedures, apparatuses that may be used, and reagent monographs. It is published every 5 years, though continual revisions take place on a regular basis. The USP also sells "reference standards" to use in determining whether substances meet USP requirements.

A sample drug monograph for acetaminophen is shown below.

Acetaminophen Monograph, Illustrated

1. Acetaminophen

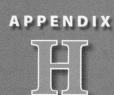

$C_8H_9NO_2$ 151.17

Acetamide, N-(4-hydroxyphenyl)-.
4'-Hydroxyacetanilide [103-90-2].

2. Acetaminophen contains not less than 98.0 percent and not more than 101.0 percent of $C_8H_9NO_2$, calculated on the anhydrous basis.

1. The monograph begins with an official title, using the *United States Adopted Name (USAN)*, as outlined under *Nomenclature <1121>*, followed by descriptive information, including a graphic formula, chemical formula, molecular weight, chemical names, and Chemical Abstracts (CAS) registry number.

2. The first item, introduced by a bold-face double-chevron symbol (>>), is the Definition. In the Definition, the content of the article is specified. It is usually given as a percentage of the chemical formula, based on the *Assay*, calculated on the anhydrous or dried basis. The assayed content of a synthetic drug substance normally should not be less than 98.0 percent and not more than 102.0 percent. The tightness of the tolerance depends on the precision of the assay used as well as on the ability to produce a drug substance of high purity without incurring unreasonable costs. For articles of lesser purity, which are derived from natural sources or fermentations, as well as for biologics (see *Biologics* <1041>), the content might be expressed in micrograms per milligram or in units per milligram.

3. Packaging and storage—Preserve in tight, light-resistant containers.

3. A discussion on packaging and storage is found in the *General Notices* under *Preservation, Packaging, Storage, and Labeling*. The proper packaging and storage conditions should be derived and documented from stability studies on the bulk drug. These standards are also important and applicable to storage and repackaging within the community pharmacy.

4. USP Reference standards <11>—*USP Acetaminophen RS.*

4. The Reference Standards section notifies the analyst of the official USP Reference Standard(s) used in the monograph and refers to the general test chapter *USP Reference Standards* <11> for additional information and instructions. Reference Standards are supplied by USP. (See also the section on *Reference Standards* in the *General Notices*).

5. *Change to read:*

5. Although technically not part of the monograph, this is a key revision phrase, which denotes that an official revision has occurred (see No. 6). The superscript black box is the beginning of the change and the subscript black box with a numeral signals the end of the change. The number at the end denotes the *Supplement* that the revision becomes official. (The official date of each *Supplement* is listed on the front cover of each *Supplement*.) Other revision phrases include *"Add the following:"* and *"Delete the following:"*

6. Identification

A: *Infrared Absorption* <197K>.

B: *Ultraviolet Absorption* <197U>—

6. Identification tests are discussed in *Procedures* under *Tests and Assays* in the *General Notices and Requirements*. They are "…provided as an aid in verifying the identity of articles. Such tests, however specific, are not necessarily sufficient to establish proof of identity…

Solution: 5 µg per mL.
Medium: 0.1 N hydrochloric acid in methanol (1 in 100).

C: It responds to the *Thin-layer Chromatographic Identification Test* <201>, a test solution in methanol containing about 1 mg per mL and a solvent system consisting of a mixture of methylene chloride and methanol (4:1) being used.

Other tests and specifications in the monograph often contribute to establishing or confirming the identity of the article under examination."

The most conclusive test for identity is the infrared absorption spectrum (see *Spectrophotometry and Light-scattering* <851>). When taken together, absorption bands characteristic of individual functional groups are unique for a given chemical compound with few exceptions. Conformance with both infrared absorption and ultraviolet absorption test specifications "leaves little doubt…regarding the identity of the specimen under examination" (see *Spectrophotometric Identification Tests* <197>). If no suitable infrared spectrum can be obtained, the *Thin-layer Chromatographic Identification Test* <201> is a good substitute. Care has to be taken to ensure that the chromatographic system separates the article from other closely related drug substances. When a drug substance is a salt, identification of the base or acid used is also provided. This is particularly important if an active principle is available in several salt forms. Identification tests for the most frequently used acids or bases can be found in *Identification Tests—General* <191>.

7. Melting range <741>: between 168° and 172°.

7. For many organic compounds the melting range or temperature is a convenient criterion of identity and purity. Generally, for a melting range to be useful it should not exceed 3° or 4°. This test should not be specified when the substance melts with decomposition; rather, such characteristics are given in *USP* in the *Reference Tables* under *Description and Solubility*.

8. Water, *Method I* <921>: not more than 0.5%.

8. If water is the only residual solvent, or if it is present as a hydrate, it must be determined for the reasons given for *Procedures* under *Tests and Assays* in the *General Notices*. *Water Determination* <921> describes the various methods that might be applicable for a given article.

9. Residue on ignition <281>: not more than 0.1%.

9. Residue on ignition can be regarded as a purity test because it limits contamination with inorganic matter (salts) in an organic compound. Such contamination would not be readily detectable by the assay, particularly a chromatographic one. It also serves as

10. Chloride <221>—Shake 1.0 g with 25 mL of water, filter, and add 1 mL of 2 N nitric acid and 1 mL of silver nitrate TS: the filtrate shows no more chloride than corresponds to 0.20 mL of 0.020 N hydrochloric acid (0.014%).

Sulfate <221>—Shake 1.0 g with 25 mL of water, filter, add 2 mL of 1 N acetic acid, then add 2 mL of barium chloride TS: the mixture shows no more sulfate than corresponds to 0.20 mL of 0.020 N sulfuric acid (0.02%).

Sulfide—Place about 2.5 g in a 50-mL beaker. Add 5 mL of alcohol and 1 mL of 3 N hydrochloric acid. Moisten a piece of lead acetate test paper with water, and fix to the underside of a watch glass. Cover the beaker with the watch glass so that part of the lead acetate paper hangs down near the pouring spout of the beaker. Heat the contents of the beaker on a hot plate just to boiling: no coloration or spotting of the test paper occurs.

11. Heavy metals, *Method II* <231>: 0.001%.

12. Free *p*-aminophenol—Transfer 5.0 g to a 100-mL volumetric flask, and dissolve in about 75 mL of a mixture of equal volumes of methanol and water. Add 5.0 mL of alkaline nitroferricyanide solution (prepared by dissolving 1 g of sodium nitroferricyanide and 1 g of anhydrous sodium carbonate in 100 mL of water), dilute with a mixture of equal volumes of methanol and water to volume, mix, and allow to stand for 30 minutes. Concomitantly determine the absorbances of this solution and of a freshly prepared solution of

an identity test for compounds with heavier inorganic counterions or inorganic functional groups.

10. These tests are provided as general procedures where limits of chloride or sulfate salts are specified.

11. This limit test, which actually determines heavy metals relative to a lead standard, should be used whenever contamination with toxic metals introduced during the manufacturing process is suspected. With modern methods of synthesis and modern supplies of acids, the need for such a test requirement seems to have lessened somewhat, at least in developed countries, and it has been possible to lower the limits for heavy metals in a number of articles.

12. Toxic impurities, arising out of the synthesis or degradation of an article, are those possessing undesirable biological properties. They must be controlled by suitable tests to a level not considered harmful. The manufacturer must notify USP concerning the presence of such impurities and should provide methods and validation data for a limit test. Suitable limit tests employ either chromatographic methods or specific and sensitive spectrophotometric and chemical methods.

p-aminophenol, similarly prepared at a concentration of 2.5 μg per mL, using the same quantities of the same reagents, in 1-cm cells, at the maximum at about 710 nm, with a suitable spectrophotometer, using 5.0 mL of alkaline nitroferricyanide solution diluted with a mixture of equal volumes of methanol and water to 100 mL as the blank: the absorbance of the test solution does not exceed that of the standard solution, corresponding to not more than 0.005% of *p*-aminophenol.

Limit of *p*-chloroacetanilide—Transfer 1.0 g to a glass-stoppered, 15-mL centrifuge tube, add 5.0 mL of ether, shake by mechanical means for 30 minutes, and centrifuge at 1000 rpm for 15 minutes or until a clean separation is obtained. Apply 200 μL of the supernatant liquid, in 40-μL portions, to obtain a single spot not more than 10 mm in diameter to a suitable thin-layer chromatographic plate (see *Chromatography* <621>) coated with a 0.25-mm layer of chromatographic silica gel mixture. Similarly apply 40 μL of a Standard solution in ether containing 10 μg of *p*-chloroacetanilide per mL, and allow the spots to dry. Develop the chromatogram in an unsaturated chamber, with a solvent system consisting of a mixture of solvent hexane and acetone (75:25), until the solvent front has moved three-fourths of the length of the plate. Remove the plate from the developing chamber, mark the solvent front, and allow the solvent to evaporate. Locate the spots in the chromatogram by examination under short-wavelength ultraviolet light: any spot obtained from the solution under test, at an R_f value corresponding to the principal spot from the Standard solution, is not greater in size or intensity than the principal spot obtained form the Standard solution, corresponding to not more than 0.001% of *p*-chloroacetanilide.

13. Readily carbonizable substances <271>— Dissolve 0.50 g in 5 mL of sulfuric acid TS: the solution has no more color than *Matching Fluid A*.

13. This nonspecific test is applied to substances that are not readily carbonized by sulfuric acid in order to limit the presence of concomitant impurities that are readily carbonized.

Change to read:

14. Organic volatile impurities, *Method V* <467>: meets the requirements.

Solvent—Use dimethyl sulfoxide as the solvent.

14. This limit test determines organic volatile impurities relative to a standard preparation containing chloroform, benzene, 1,2-dioxane, methylene chloride, and trichloroethylene. The limits are 50, 100, 100, 500, and 1,000 ppm, respectively. The test is required for bulk substances and excipients that are used in chronic-systemic administered dosage forms. The three main analytical methods used are based on the use of gas chromatography.

15. Assay—Dissolve about 120 mg of Acetaminophen, accurately weighed, in 10 mL of methanol in a 500-mL volumetric flask, dilute with water to volume, and mix. Transfer 5.0 mL of this solution to a 100-mL volumetric flask, dilute with water to volume, and mix. Concomitantly determine the absorbances of this solution and of a Standard solution of USP Acetaminophen RS, in the same medium, at a concentration of about 12 µg per mL in 1-cm cells, at the wavelength of maximum absorbance at about 244 nm, with a suitable spectrophotometer, using water as the blank. Calculate the quantity, in mg, of $C_8H_9NO_2$ in the Acetaminophen taken by the formula:

$10C(A_U/A_S)$, in which C is the concentration in m g per mL, of USP Acetaminophen RS in the Standard solution, and A_U and A_S are the absorbances of the solution of Acetaminophen and the Standard solution, respectively.

15. Tolerances in the Definition are based on the *Assay*. They, therefore, should be as precise as possible. The *Assay* does not have to be stability-indicating, but the monograph, taken as a whole, should assure that any degradation would be detected and can be limited by a chromatographic or other specific test. An ideal combination is a chromatographic test for ordinary impurities with a precise titrimetric assay. Microbial assays for antibiotics (see *Antibiotics— Microbial Assays* <81>) are currently replaced by HPLC (see *Chromatography* <621>) assays, wherever possible. However, for antibiotics that are mixtures of several active components, the microbial assay is still the preferred one and is sometimes coupled with a chromatographic test to quantitate the individual components. Biologics, proteins, and peptides may require very specialized biological assays.

* *The explanations of each of the monograph sections are based on an article that appeared in the* Pharmacopeial Forum *Vol. 15 No. 5, A Guide to USP Standards by Klaus G. Florey, Ph.D. Dr. Florey was a member of the USP Committee of Revision from 1970 to 1995.*

Glossary

A

Administrative law – The body of law governing the administrative agencies (e.g., Occupational Safety and Health Administration or the Department of Public Health) that have been created by Congress or by state legislatures.

Adulteration – Tampering with or contaminating a product or substance.

Airflow hood – A workstation that emits a stream of highly filtered air that reduces possible contamination of the substances being used.

Anabolic steroids – Schedule III controlled substances (either drugs or hormonal substances) that are often misused by athletes seeking to enhance their bulk (by increasing muscle mass) and physical prowess.

Appeal – A legal process in which a case is brought to a higher court to review the decision of a lower court.

Autonomy – The ability or tendency to function independently.

Auxiliary labels – Labels applied to drug containers that supply additional information, such as whether to take the medication with or without food, potential adverse effects, to avoid taking with alcohol, etc.

B

Biohazard symbol – An international symbol that is used to designate any substance harmful to human health, including bloodborne pathogens and medical wastes.

Bloodborne pathogen – Any infectious microorganism present in blood or other body fluids and tissues.

C

"C" symbol – A marking that indicates a controlled substance, and is printed on a drug's label, its box, and/or its packaging insert.

Case law – A system of law based on judges' decisions and legal precedents rather than on statutes; in this system, judges can interpret statutory law or apply common law.

Chemical hygiene plan – A "laboratory standard" established by OSHA to reduce exposures to chemicals when handled by employees.

Code of ethics – Standards developed to affect quality and ensure the highest ethical and professional behavior.

Common law – A system of law derived from the decisions of judges rather than from constitutions or statutes.

Compensation claim – A claim filed with the state that addresses an onsite workplace injury or illness.

Compliance program guidelines – HIPAA-related privacy, training, and security regulations designed to focus on, correct, and maintain good health-care practices.

Continuing education – Instructional learning that keeps an individual up-to-date with advancements in their field.

Contract law – A system of law that pertains to agreements between two or more parties.

Criminal law – The body of law that defines criminal offenses against the public.

D

Data processing system – An alternative, computerized method for the storage and retrieval of prescription refill information for controlled substances in Schedules III and IV.

DEA number – A series of numbers assigned to a health-care practitioner that allows him or her to write prescriptions for controlled substances.

Disclosure – Transferring information, releasing information, providing access to information, or divulging information in any manner.

Down time – A period of time when a computer or computer system is not operational, for any of a variety of reasons.

Drug Enforcement Administration (DEA) – The bureau within the United States Department of Justice primarily responsible for policing federal laws that concern controlled substances. In addition to investigating the sellers, producers, and smugglers of illicit drugs, the DEA also monitors physician prescribing patterns and pharmacy purchases.

Drug history – A history of a patient's medication use over a reasonable period of time, usually for at least the last 5 years; it includes all documented information on prescription medications, non-prescription (OTC) medications, and supplements.

E

Electronic data interchange (EDI) – A set of standards for structuring electronic information intended to be exchanged between different entities.

Electronic medical records (EMR) – Preferred method of record storage (over paper records) because their electronic format can be accessed more quickly and takes less room to store.

Encryption – Transforming information via an algorithm to make it unreadable to anyone who does not possess the decryption information required to read it.

Ethics – The study of value, or morals and morality; it includes concepts such as right, wrong, good, evil, and responsibility.

Extranet – A private network that uses Internet protocols, network connections, and sometimes telecommunication devices to share information with outside entities.

F

Facsimile – A copy of an official document (such as a prescription or medication order) that is commonly transmitted via fax machine.

Fax paper – A special paper that burns a thermal image of a transmitted document without using regular paper and printer ink or toner; this type of paper usually causes the burned text and/or images to fade over time.

Federal Register – A U.S. government publication that contains all administrative laws, and is the primary source of information for OSHA standards.

Felony – An offense punishable by imprisonment or death in a state or federal prison for more than one year.

Fire safety plan – A workplace plan detailing locations of fire alarm pull boxes, fire extinguishers, and fire sprinklers, as well as a plan for continued fire prevention training and drills.

Fraud – The intentional use of deceit to deprive another person of his or her money, property, or rights.

Fraudulent – Deceitful; intending to deceive.

G

Germicides – Agents that kill germs, also known as "disinfectants."

H

Hazard communication plan – A system of notifying personnel of hazards by applying warning labels that signify the types and ratings of hazardous chemicals and substances.

Hazardous waste – A solid, chemical, radioactive, or infectious material that may transmit pathogens or other hazardous substances.

I

Infringements – Violations of laws, regulations, or agreements.

Investigational – Drugs used to provide detailed inquiry or systematic examination of their effects.

J

Jurisdiction – The power and authority given to a court to hear a case and to make a judgment.

L

Law – A rule of conduct or procedure established by custom, agreement, or authority.

Legal precedent – A legal principle created by a court decision that provides an example for judges deciding similar issues later.

Legend drug – Prescription drug.

Legislative law – A law that is prescribed by legislative enactments; also known as statutory law.

Licensure – The practice of granting professional licenses to practice a profession.

Loyalty – A faithfulness or allegiance to a cause, ideal, custom, institution, or product.

M

Magistrates – Civil officers with the power to enforce laws.

Malfeasance – The execution of an unlawful or improper act.

Malpractice – Professional misconduct or demonstration of an unreasonable lack of skill with the result of injury, loss, or damage to the patient.

Material Safety Data Sheet (MSDS) – A form that is required for all hazardous chemicals or other substances that are used in laboratories or pharmacies. This form contains information about a product's name, chemical characteristics, ingredients, guidelines for safe handling, physical and health hazards, and procedures to be followed in the event of exposure.

Medical code sets – Sets of alphanumeric codes used for encoding medical conditions, diseases, procedures, and other information.

Medical Waste Tracking Act – An act that gives OSHA the authority to inspect hazardous medical waste and cite offices for unhealthy or unsafe practices regarding them.

Misbranding – Fraudulent or misleading labeling or marking.

Misdemeanor – Crimes punishable by fine or by imprisonment in a facility other than a prison for less than one year.

Misfeasance – The improper performance of an act.

Morals – Motivations based on ideas of right and wrong.

N

National Drug Code (NDC) – The federal code that identifies a drug's manufacturer or distributor, its formulation, and the size and type of its packaging.

National Formulary (NF) standards – Standards concerning medicines, dosage forms, drug substances, excipients (inactive substances used as carriers for active medicinal ingredients), medical devices, and dietary supplements.

NDC number – A product identifier used for drugs intended for human use; "NDC" stands for "National Drug Code."

Negligence – A type of unintentional tort alleged when one may have performed or failed to perform an act that a reasonable person would or would not have done in similar circumstances.

Nonfeasance – The failure to act when there is a duty to act, as a reasonably prudent person would in similar circumstances.

Notice of Privacy Practices (NOPP) – A document that explains to patients how his or her PHI may be used and disclosed.

O

Occupational Safety and Health Administration (OSHA) – A division of the U.S. Department of Labor.

Office of the Inspector General (OIG) – Governmental office that investigates various organizations, including health-care organizations, to assure integrity and efficiency in their operations.

Orphan drug – Drugs used to treat diseases that affect fewer than 200,000 people in the United States.

Over-the-counter (OTC) – Non-prescription drug.

P

Pharmacy compounding – Creating a new mixture or compound by blending or mixing two or more medications and other substances in a licensed pharmacy.

Pharmacy internship – A period of service in a pharmacy, wherein a pharmacy student works, under supervision, to gain practical experience.

Phocomelia – A severe birth defect also known as "seal limbs," involving the malformation or non-formation of arms and legs; it was caused by the drug thalidomide.

Professional ethics – Moral standards and principles of conduct guiding professionals in performing their functions.

Prosecution – A legal proceeding against an individual.

Protected Health Information (PHI) – All stored health information that relates to a past, present, or future physical or mental health condition.

R

Radioactive waste – Any waste that contains or is contaminated with liquid or solid radioactive materials.

Revocation – Recall of authority or power to act.

Revoked – Voided, annulled, recalled, withdrawn, or reversed.

S

Schedules – The five classifications of controlled substances, with the drugs having the highest potential for abuse and no medical use listed in Schedule I, and those with progressively less abuse potential listed in Schedules II, III, IV, and V.

Security Rule – A HIPAA-related regulation that specifies how PHI is protected on computer networks, the Internet, the extranet, and disks and other storage media.

Statute of limitations – That period of time established by state law during which a lawsuit or criminal proceeding may be filed.

Statutory law – A law that is prescribed by legislative enactments; also known as legislative law.

T

Teratogenic – Causing genetic defects.

Tort – A private wrong or injury, other than a breach of contract, for which the court will provide a remedy.

Treatment, payment, and health care operations (TPHCO) – This concerns PHI that may be shared in order to provide treatment, process payment, and operate the medical business.

U

United States Pharmacopoeia (USP) – The officially recognized authority and standard on the prescription of drugs, chemicals, and medicinal preparations in the United States.

V

Values – Desirable standards or qualities.

W

Workers' compensation – Laws that establish procedures for compensating workers who are injured on the job, with the employer paying the cost of the insurance premium for the employee.

Index